Demons in the Consulting Room

Demons in the Consulting Room: Echoes of genocide, slavery and extreme trauma in psychoanalytic practice is the second of two volumes addressing the overwhelming, often unmetabolizable feelings related to mourning, both on an individual and mass scale. Authors in this volume explore the potency of ghosts, ghostliness, and the darker, often grotesque aspects of these phenomena. While ghosts can be spectral presences that we feel protective of, demons haunt in a particularly virulent way, distorting experience, our sense of reality, and our character.

Bringing together a collection of clinical and theoretical papers, *Demons in the Consulting Room* reveals how the most extreme types of trauma can continue to have effects across generations, and how these effects manifest in the consulting room. Essays in this volume consider traumas that have affected multiple generations of people, such as the Holocaust, experiences in the gulags, and the experience of slavery. Authors here consider the clinical challenges of working with the demonic force in severe childhood abuse and the effects of serious and prolonged physical injury and illness. Inevitably, there is in such difficult clinical work the combined effects of hauntings in the analysts and in patients and often in the surrounding culture.

In this book, distinguished psychoanalysts explore the myriad forms of ghosts and the demonic, which interfere and disrupt the endlessly difficult psychic work of mourning. It will be of interest to psychotherapists and psychoanalysts, as well as social workers, family therapists, psychologists, and psychiatrists. *Demons in the Consulting Room* will appeal to those specializing in bereavement and trauma and, on a broader level, to sociologists and historians interested in understanding means of coping with loss and grief on both an individual and larger scale basis.

Adrienne Harris is on the faculty and is a supervisor at the NYU Postdoctoral Program in Psychotherapy and Psychoanalysis. She published *Gender as Soft Assembly* in 2005. She writes about gender and development, about analytic subjectivity, and about the analysts developing and writing around the period of the First World War.

Margery Kalb is a psychologist and psychoanalyst in private practice in New York City. She is on the faculty at the NYU Postdoctoral Program in Psychotherapy and Psychoanalysis. She also teaches and supervises clinical work for the doctoral psychology program at Pace University. Dr. Kalb is the author of several papers on ghosts.

Susan Klebanoff is a clinical psychologist and psychoanalyst in private practice in New York City. She is on the faculty of the Stephen Mitchell Center and is an adjunct clinical supervisor at the Ferkauf School of Yeshiva University. Klebanoff has previously co-authored a book on depression for middle school aged children and a chapter in a book on uncertainty in psychoanalysis.

RELATIONAL PERSPECTIVES BOOK SERIES

LEWIS ARON & ADRIENNE HARRIS
Series Co-Editors

STEVEN KUCHUCK & EYAL ROZMARIN
Associate Editors

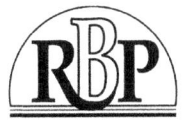

The Relational Perspectives Book Series (RPBS) publishes books that grow out of or contribute to the relational tradition in contemporary psychoanalysis. The term *relational psychoanalysis* was first used by Greenberg and Mitchell[1] to bridge the traditions of interpersonal relations, as developed within interpersonal psychoanalysis and object relations, as developed within contemporary British theory. But, under the seminal work of the late Stephen Mitchell, the term *relational psychoanalysis* grew and began to accrue to itself many other influences and developments. Various tributaries—interpersonal psychoanalysis, object relations theory, self psychology, empirical infancy research, and elements of contemporary Freudian and Kleinian thought—flow into this tradition, which understands relational configurations between self and others, both real and fantasied, as the primary subject of psychoanalytic investigation.

We refer to the relational tradition, rather than to a relational school, to highlight that we are identifying a trend, a tendency within contemporary psychoanalysis, not a more formally organized or coherent school or system of beliefs. Our use of the term *relational* signifies a dimension of theory and practice that has become salient across the wide spectrum of contemporary psychoanalysis. Now under the editorial supervision of Lewis Aron and Adrienne Harris with the assistance of Associate Editors Steven Kuchuck and Eyal Rozmarin, the Relational Perspectives Book Series originated in 1990 under the editorial eye of the late Stephen A. Mitchell.

1 Greenberg, J. & Mitchell, S. (1983). *Object relations in psychoanalytic theory.* Cambridge, MA: Harvard University Press.

Mitchell was the most prolific and influential of the originators of the relational tradition. He was committed to dialogue among psychoanalysts and he abhorred the authoritarianism that dictated adherence to a rigid set of beliefs or technical restrictions. He championed open discussion, comparative and integrative approaches, and he promoted new voices across the generations.

Included in the Relational Perspectives Book Series are authors and works that come from within the relational tradition, extend and develop the tradition, as well as works that critique relational approaches or compare and contrast it with alternative points of view. The series includes our most distinguished senior psychoanalysts, along with younger contributors who bring fresh vision.

A full list of titles in this series is available at https://www.routledge.com/series/LEARPBS. Recently published titles:

Vol. 69
Relational Treatment of Trauma: Stories of Loss and Hope
Toni Heineman

Vol. 70
Freud's Legacy in the Global Era
Carlo Strenger

Vol. 71
The Enigma of Desire: Sex, Longing, and Belonging in Psychoanalysis
Galit Atlas

Vol. 72
Conservative and Radical Perspectives on Psychoanalytic Knowledge: The Fascinated and the Disenchanted
Aner Govrin

Vol. 73
Immigration in Psychoanalysis: Locating Ourselves
Julia Beltsiou

Vol. 74
The Dissociative Mind in Psychoanalysis: Understanding and Working With Trauma
Elizabeth Howell & Sheldon Itzkowitz

Vol. 75
Ghosts in the Consulting Room: Echoes of Trauma in Psychoanalysis
Adrienne Harris, Margery Kalb and Susan Klebanoff

Vol. 76
Demons in the Consulting Room: Echoes of Genocide, Slavery and Extreme Trauma in Psychoanalytic Practice
Adrienne Harris, Margery Kalb and Susan Klebanoff

Vol. 77
The Ethical Turn: Otherness and Subjectivity in Contemporary Psychoanalysis
David M. Goodman and Eric R. Severson

Demons in the Consulting Room

Echoes of genocide, slavery, and extreme trauma in psychoanalytic practice

Edited by Adrienne Harris, Margery Kalb, and Susan Klebanoff

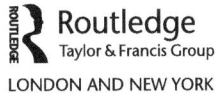

LONDON AND NEW YORK

In memory of Muriel Dimen (1942–2016)

First published 2017
by Routledge
2 Park Square, Milton Park, Abingdon, Oxon OX14 4RN

and by Routledge
711 Third Avenue, New York, NY 10017

Routledge is an imprint of the Taylor & Francis Group, an informa business

© 2017 selection and editorial matter, Adrienne Harris, Margery Kalb, Susan Klebanoff; individual chapters, the contributors

The right of the editors to be identified as the authors of the editorial material, and of the authors for their individual chapters, has been asserted in accordance with sections 77 and 78 of the Copyright, Designs and Patents Act 1988.

All rights reserved. No part of this book may be reprinted or reproduced or utilised in any form or by any electronic, mechanical, or other means, now known or hereafter invented, including photocopying and recording, or in any information storage or retrieval system, without permission in writing from the publishers.

Trademark notice: Product or corporate names may be trademarks or registered trademarks, and are used only for identification and explanation without intent to infringe.

British Library Cataloguing in Publication Data
A catalogue record for this book is available from the British Library

Library of Congress Cataloging in Publication Data
Names: Harris, Adrienne, editor. | Kalb, Margery, editor. | Klebanoff, Susan, editor.
Title: Demons in the consulting room : echoes of genocide, slavery and extreme trauma in psychoanalytic practice / edited by Adrienne Harris, Margery Kalb and Susan Klebanoff.
Description: Hove, East Sussex ; New York, NY : Routledge, 2016.
Identifiers: LCCN 2015044119| ISBN 9781138943483 (hbk) | ISBN 9781138943490 (pbk)
Subjects: LCSH: Psychic trauma. | Grief. | Psychoanalysis.
Classification: LCC BF175.5.P75 D46 2016 | DDC 155.9/3—dc23
LC record available at http://lccn.loc.gov/2015044119

ISBN: 978-1-138-94348-3 (hbk)
ISBN: 978-1-138-94349-0 (pbk)
ISBN: 978-1-315-67241-0 (ebk)

Typeset in Times New Roman
by Swales & Willis Ltd, Exeter, Devon, UK

Contents

List of figures	ix
Author biographies	x
Introduction ADRIENNE HARRIS, MARGERY KALB, AND SUSAN KLEBANOFF	1

Clinical 17

1	Ghosts in the consulting room: reluctant ancestors MARGERY KALB	19
2	The Dybbuk: it's me or him GALIT ATLAS	46
3	Occupation: a ghost story ARTHUR FOX	59
4	Repressed ghosts and dissociated vampires in the enacted dimension of psychoanalytic treatment GIL KATZ	69
5	Do we find or lose ourselves in the negative? JADE MCGLEUGHLIN	93

Community & culture 123

6	The past is the presence between us: psychoanalysis and the specter of the Shoah EMILY A. KURILOFF	125

7	Ghosts and the sexual boundary violation: the limits of an idea MURIEL DIMEN	140
8	Basic uncertainty and totalitarian objects MICHAEL ŠEBEK	148
9	The presence of the past: transmission of slavery's traumas JANICE P. GUMP	159
10	Wounded stories ALEXANDER ETKIND	179
	Afterword SAM GERSON	198
	Index	203

Figures

5.1	Polka Dots, Providence, Rhode Island. Courtesy of George and Betty Woodman	102
5.2	Space, Providence, Rhode Island 1976. Courtesy of George and Betty Woodman	104
5.3	About Being My Model, Providence 1976. Courtesy of George and Betty Woodman	105
5.4	Untitled, Providence 1976. Courtesy of George and Betty Woodman	106
5.5	Untitled, Boulder Colorado 1972–1975. Courtesy of George and Betty Woodman	107
5.6	Untitled, Rome 1977–1978. Courtesy of George and Betty Woodman	110

Author biographies

Galit Atlas is a psychoanalyst and clinical supervisor in private practice in New York City. She is a member of the faculty at the NYU Postdoctoral Program in Psychotherapy and Psychoanalysis, the Four Year Adult and National Training Programs at NIP, and the Institute for Expressive Analysis. She serves on the editorial board of *Psychoanalytic Perspectives*, is on the board of directors of the Division (39) of psychoanalysis, APA, and is the author of articles and book chapters that focus primarily on gender and sexuality. Her book *The Enigma of Desire-Sex, Longing and Belonging in Psychoanalysis* is published as part of Routledge's Relational Perspectives Book Series.

Muriel Dimen, Ph.D. was Adjunct Clinical Professor, Psychology, at NYU Postdoctoral Program Psychotherapy and Psychoanalysis and Professor Emerita, Anthropology, Lehman. She was Editor-in-Chief of *Studies Gend. Sex.*, associate editor of, *Psych. Dial.*; founder, IARPP. Editor, *With Culture in Mind* (Routledge, 2011). Her books include *Sexuality, Intimacy, Power* (Analytic Press, 2003, Goethe Award, Canadian Psychological Association); *Surviving Sexual Contradictions* (Macmillan, 1986); *The Anthropological Imagination* (McGraw-Hill, 1977). She is co-editor of the following books: *Gender in Psychoanalytic Space* (with V. Goldner, Other Press, 2002); *Storms in Her Head* (with A. Harris. Other Press, 2001); *Regional Variation Modern Greece and Cyprus* (with E. Friedl, NY Academy of Sciences 263, 1976). She is a fellow, of the NY Institute for Humanities, NYU.

Alexander Etkind is Professor of History at the European University Institute at Florence. He has just moved to EUI after many years of teaching as professor at the University of Cambridge, where he was also a fellow at King's College. Etkind was born in St. Petersburg and defended his Ph.D. in Helsinki. He is the author of *Eros of the Impossible. The History of Psychoanalysis in Russia* (Westview Press, 1996); *Internal Colonization: Russia's Imperial Experience* (Polity Press, 2011); and *Warped Mourning: Stories of the Undead in the Land of the Unburied* (Stanford University Press, 2013). He also co-edited *Memory and Theory in Eastern Europe* (Palgrave, 2013) and co-authored *Remembering Katyn* (Polity, 2012). His most recent project is an intellectual biography of William Bullitt, first American ambassador to Soviet Russia.

Arthur Fox, Ph.D., trained in psychoanalysis at the NYU Postdoctoral Program, and at the City University of New York. He is an adjunct clinical supervisor at CUNY and teaches at the Manhattan Institute for Psychoanalysis. He is in private practice in New York City.

Sam Gerson, Ph.D., is a founder, past-president, and a training and supervising analyst at the Psychoanalytic Institute of Northern California. *In 2007 h*e received the Elise M. Hayman Award for the Study of Genocide and the Holocaust from the International Psychoanalytic Association for his paper entitled "When the Third is Dead: Memory, Mourning and Witnessing in the Aftermath of the Holocaust"; published in the *International Journal of Psychoanalysis* in 2009. At the IPA Congress in Prague in 2013 he presented "Mourning and Melancholia After the Holocaust: A Psychoanalytic Exploration of the Suicides of Jean Amery, Paul Celan, and Primo Levi".

Janice P. Gump, Ph.D., is in private practice in Washington DC and a member of the Institute of Contemporary Psychotherapy & Psychoanalysis. She has been a faculty member of the Howard University Medical School and Psychology Department, as well as the Washington School of Psychiatry. She has also been a consulting editor for the *Journal of Consulting and Clinical Psychology*, a reviewer for the Mental Health Small Grants Committee, NIMH, and a member of the Professional Psychology Editorial Board. Dr. Gump has authored papers on African American women, shame, and the enduring consequences of slavery's traumas upon African American subjectivity.

Margery Kalb is a psychologist, psychoanalyst, and supervisor in private practice in New York City. She is on the faculty of the NYU Postdoctoral Program in Psychotherapy and Psychoanalysis (Clinical Assistant Professor of Psychology), where she teaches a course entitled *Ghosts in the Consulting Room: A Clinical Seminar on Repetitive (Re)Enactments*. She also teaches clinical case seminars and supervises individual clinical work for the doctoral psychology program at Pace University. She is the author of several papers on ghosts, encompassing themes such as transference-countertransference, somatization, anxiety, values/morality, loss, and mourning.

Gil Katz, Ph.D., is a clinical associate professor of psychology, faculty member, and supervising analyst in the Contemporary Freudian Track of the NYU Postdoctoral Program in Psychotherapy and Psychoanalysis, and faculty member, training analyst, and former Dean of Training at the Institute for Psychoanalytic Training and Research. He teaches courses on interaction and enactment in psychoanalysis at both institutes. Dr. Katz has written widely on the topic of enactment, most recently a book entitled: *The Play within the Play: The Enacted Dimension of Psychoanalytic Process*. He has also written on such subjects as the analytic usefulness of working within the metaphor, the parallel process phenomenon in analytic supervision, and analytic understandings of father-son rivalry in biblical tales. He is in private practice in Manhattan.

Emily A. Kuriloff, Psy.D., is a clinical psychologist, training and supervising analyst at the William Alanson White Institute, where she is also the Director of Clinical Education. She is the former Book Review Editor, and current Outreach Editor for the journal, *Contemporary Psychoanalysis*. Dr. Kuriloff has written numerous articles and book chapters exploring the history of psychoanalysis, and comparative models of therapeutic action and praxis. Her current book, *Contemporary Psychoanalysis and the Legacy of the Third Reich; History, Memory and Tradition* was published by Routledge in 2014.

Jade McGleughlin, L.I.C.S.W., is a supervising and personal analyst, supervisor, faculty member, board member at, and president elect The Massachusetts Institute For Psychoanalysis. She is on the editorial boards of *Psychoanalytic Dialogues* and *Studies in Gender and Sexuality*. Her most recent papers on this topic are, "Do We Lose Ourselves in the Negative", and Answering Gestures April 2015 and "The Analyst's Necessary Vertigo", September 2011, each in *Psychoanalytic Dialogues*. She is in private practice in Cambridge MA in psychoanalysis/psychotherapy/supervision and consultation to difficult therapies. She sees both children and adults.

Michael Šebek, Ph.D., CSc., is a training and supervising analyst at the Czech Psychoanalytic Society, former president twice elected, former director of the Psychoanalytic Institute of the Czech Psychoanalytical Society, former member of the international board of the journal *Psychoanalytic Inquiry* (1993–2010), secretary of the IPA President D. Widlocher for Europe (2000–2002), And Erikson Scholar of the Erikson Institute of the Austen Riggs Center in Stockbridge, MA in 1999. Since 1995 he has carried out training activities for the Han Groen Prakken Institute for Eastern Europe and since 2013 has been a member of the Sponsoring Committee of the IPA for the Moscow Group of Psychoanalysis.

Introduction

Adrienne Harris, Margery Kalb, and Susan Klebanoff

This book and its companion, edited collections of essays on "ghostliness" in psychoanalytic and cultural life, emerged from the collective work of a group of analysts. Both collaboratively and individually, we were struck by the way uncanny and spectral presence, or absent presence, entered minds, bodies, and consulting rooms. The attention to ghosts did not stop just in the clinical dyad. We found ghosts haunting our theories, our practices, and our training institutes. We found them in many interstices of cultural and social life, too. There is no dearth of spectral presences. In addition to familial, intrapsychic, and relational ghosts, ghosts emerge from war and catastrophes that cannot easily be assimilated in the surrounding cultures and communities or in the minds and bodies of individuals.

Ghosts emerge in and as unwitnessed silences, and surely, from actual deaths. The body may be the absorber and also the communicator of ghosts. We draw on the term "ghosts" to capture the sense of objects that are neither internal nor external solely, that may disturb the atmosphere, the soma, the mind, temporality and the surrounding fields.

We came to this topic unexpectedly. Or should we say, uncannily. We,[1] are seven psychoanalysts, different in backgrounds and in formation, who came together to discuss clinical work. The group formed out of the supervisory experience of one member and was made up of people new to each other, if not new to Adrienne Harris who formed the group.

We began a group process by reading Sam Gerson's "When the Third is Dead", (2009) his prize-winning essay on witnessing and its vicissitudes. The paper focuses on the oddness of how historic injuries accrue around, between, and within persons as "present absences." Gerson was concerned with what happens culturally and personally when there is no registration of a catastrophe that has happened, is happening, seems always already to be happening. He was interested in bearing witness and he was also interested in what happened when such witnessing failed, when registration becomes beyond the capacity of an individual or the collective. He has written afterwords to both these books, a mark for us of expanding influence on how we understand witnessing loss and its absence or failure or destruction.

Gerson deploys an evocative term for this lack of registration, "present absences." This concept appears in the work of Bollas (1994), Caruth (1996), and Ogden (1992). This phrase has been a guiding force in our group work. "Present absences" refer to just that—absences that can be emotionally, viscerally or even unconsciously felt in the patient, in the analyst, and in their interaction. These present absences grow from overwhelming but under-processed feelings about loss (frequently, though not necessarily, an actual death), and often emerge in gaps in factual information, narrative or affect—things mysteriously missing. We can think of this un-knowledge as a perpetual struggle between mourning and melancholia (Freud, 1917), something is, under wraps, a secret too dangerous to be disturbed and thus oftentimes discovered in the enacted sphere of the transference/countertransference matrix.

Reading Gerson was a way to begin a group process. This was thought of just in a rather instrumental way. We picked a common task, thinking that such common work binds people, but we must hold and ponder the question of uncanny prescience in making such a transformative choice.

The Gerson paper stimulated many interesting associations and clinical concerns in the group and, as the cases began to pile up, so too did bodies, losses—conscious and unconscious, deep uncertainties, intergenerational transmissions of trauma and, we all came to agree, ghosts. And, in a way that certainly marked the group and helped our collective and internal growth, there have been, over six years, four staggeringly difficult deaths experienced by members in the group, and the demands of serious illnesses carried privately and also borne by everyone. We have also had two weddings, joyous occasions carrying their own ghosts as well.

We offer these personal details because we suspect that they are not really very atypical. Part of the work on analytic subjectivity has been to comprehend the complexity of the interrelationship of the use of the analytic instrument and the demands of daily life (Deutsch, 2014; Harris and Sinsheimer, 2008). A commitment to a field, to a bi-personal unconscious and conscious transmission across the analytic dyad requires that we widen our view as to what enters and affects the analytic process. In the processing of the personal and the clinical, the theoretical and the historical, we were also able to, and really needed to, include our own histories and countertransferences in our group process and in our individual clinical work.

Our hope is that in the clinical work we did on ghostly presences in treatments, and in the writing it is stimulating, we can find ways to talk and think about the manner we and patients are haunted, and how these hauntings might be imagined and transformed. How do such possessions highjack lives and often treatments? Where are there demons? Are there good ghosts? Even as the presence of ghosts has historically signified the presence of unmetabolizable loss, are there limits to mourning? Is mourning to some extent an idealization, and specters grim or wistful inevitable legacies of loss?

As the group's project has evolved to include an expanded group of authors, we ask and have been asked. Why ghosts? Why demons? Why not internal objects, why not dissociation or disavowal? Why do we need this new/old perhaps, melodramatic, language? In evolving answers to these questions, are we struggling towards a new conception that lives liminally in different sectors of clinical life, cultural thought, and practices?

Theorists have thought of these phenomena differently: intergenerational transmission of trauma (Davoine, 2007; Davoine and Gaudilliere, 2004), telescoping of generations (Faimberg, 2004), witnessing and Thirdness (Benjamin, 2004; Gerson, 2009), encrypted identifications (Abraham and Torok, 1994) or radioactive identifications (Gampel, 1992; Puget, 1989, 2002). Freud, Loewald, and more contemporaneously Reis (2011) and Grand (2010) have written about the impactful presence of ghosts, vampires, and other kinds of haunting objects that enter the analytic field.

Working on ghosts and demons required an expansion of vocabulary and imagination. There are ghosts that protect, that hold us hostage; ghosts that we protect and cannot separate from (Baranger and Baranger, 2009). But there is a murderous side to this; demons and vampires, dybbuks, and monstrous and grotesque forms that often represent the impossibility of containing and metabolizing loss and trauma. The body and the mind can be the site of attack and invasion. Eros and Thanatos can intermingle and disturb individuals and cultures.

In this book we hope to explore the actual and psychic legacy of loss, of violence, phobic hatreds, and migrations that bear so heavily on the lives, minds and bodies of contemporary patients. In tracking the present-absence and absent-presence of ghosts and various forms of hauntings within psychoanalytic treatments, we are tracking the power of hidden and often shame-laden histories to enter and shape the clinical work.

You could think of the ghost world as the place to manage excess, to find a skin of strangeness and uncertainty in which to imbed things hard to bear or hard to fathom. This is another melancholy solution but rich and engaging also. In some of the chapters, particularly the clinical ones, we have found ourselves in deep engagement with the differences and meanings of melancholy and mourning, ultimately wanting to expand the space and scope and duration of melancholy, while not avoiding or reifying its pathological aspects.

Harris (2013) wrote about Bion's well-known ideas about death in life in the context of his advice to analysts to work without memory or desire.

> This is Bion's famous instruction to the analyst: work in the present moment, without reference to history and desire.
> (Bion, 1967, p. 612)

As a sentence, an invocation, a call, this sentence is charming, evocative, interesting, putting us in touch with the foundational Freudian injunction of "evenly hovering attention." Yet, we might remember Racker's reworking of this injunction as a call to meditative states, states of altered consciousness. And we also can evoke now Ferro's idea of the task of analysis as one of inducing dreaming. It is a goal of analytic work to arrive at primary process. All these ideas seem to me exceedingly useful injunctions to analysts, pushing us to be attuned to bodies, minds, affects and to try (never fully successfully) to entertain experiences "outside the sentence" (Barthes, 1975).

But let me introduce another Bion quote to add to the complexity of Bion's relationship to temporality. To wit:

> I died on August 7th, 1917, on the Amiens-Roye Road.
> (Bion 1982, p. 265)

He meant it.

So, Bion, in every waking minute, including the careful unfolding minutes of analytic sessions, is both changing, remembering, and still walking on that road, where his friend is still, in every present minute, being killed and he (Bion) not moving, or saving, or helping. And so forever, walking and dying on that road, both men. And, if so, we might say that the living man (Bion) is actually then conducting analyses from what Francoise Davoine (2007) refers to as "the bridge world," a space between the living and the dead" (Harris, 2013).

Bion was haunted, surely, but his haunting underwrote his vocation. Looked at from this biographical perspective, then, working with no history and no future, is actually at base the work of a traumatized, ghost-riddled analyst, a person working with time suspended, usefully and tragically. This might be so for all of us, even if our traumas are significantly less acute than Bion's. Loewald, (1989) too, talks about this and so we might include him in this account of the impact of trauma on theory building, wondering what was carried personally for him, from the death of his father and the bereavement of his mother, in the injunction to turn a ghost into an ancestor.

Here is another Bion notion. Patients and analysts are working always at the edge of the abyss, the terror at the moments of transition (Goldberg, 2008). James Grotstein, Bion's analysand, thinks that Bion remained stymied, stuck, hopelessly lost in the wake of the death of that beloved friend in 1917. Grotstein ends his discussion of Bion's memoir with this comment:

> Someone once said that Bion was "miles behind his face." I take this to mean that he was withdrawn, lonely, and unreached.
> (Grotstein, 1998, p. 613)

If you are a psychoanalyst caught up in this way of seeing the task or problem of analysis, history is necessary but history is an albatross. Sometimes the ghostliness seems embodied in spectral presences, in figures actually dead or missing. Fascinating psychic processes underlie the deeply committed attempts patients make to keep the dead alive, close down space, or alternatively keep it open and ready for habitation. Killing and saving seem often too close to each other.

Rey (1988) has an intriguing way of thinking about this: the task of the analysand is to have the analyst cure the damaged objects he/she brings to the work. And, as Harris (2009) has argued, in clinical impasses, we often see how the analyst similarly arrives in the work to cure old injuries, bury the undead, undertake the final repair of history.

The task of repair of internal objects, laced into our countertransferences, is the source and wellspring of powerful sublimations and transformations into work ethics and skill. But there remains in anyone conducting this work, the residue of uneasy spirits and unfixed figures. Part of the shared task of analytic work is the transformation of melancholy into mourning, an always partially incomplete task. Many chapters in this book attest to the unending exhausting task of mourning. Margaret Little's pronouncement seems apt, "Mourning is for life" (Little, M, 1985).

It was in considering our clinical work and the complexity of encryption that we found it necessary to consider the profound role of the body and embodiment. In the current theoretical work on reconsidering levels of representation and registration of experience (Botella and Botella, 2005; Levine, Reed, and Scarfone, 2013; Stern, 2015) we are reaching for an account of what the body carries and communicates that builds on different models of mind and body, more integrated ideas of mental and bodily life and the complex structures in which experience is carried. As variable phenomena as body image, somatic illnesses, affect storms, gait, posture, the set of the face and gaze, the experience of weather, of space and time, are all saturated in meaning. Indeed, each and every one of our clinical chapters encompasses some form of unstable somatic dimensions. We have found it useful to see these phenomena as ghostly, spectral, and ambiguous.

Although we began in the consulting room we found we could not entirely stay there. In many traditional cultures, ghosts and the spirit world can live both easily and strangely within daily life. Looking back now, it is fascinating to realize that the popular culture following the First World War seemed full of ghosts and vampires, creatures popping out of movies and television and popular novels. Was this popular depiction an attempt to contain or perhaps express the cultural level of melancholy and mourning? Did these effects and influences come from the past (slavery, wars, historical trauma, gulags) or, as some might say, from the future already present (climate change, terrorism, economic pain)?

In thinking of the long shadow of war (in both familial and cultural intergenerational transmission of trauma), we encountered some other interesting material on ghosts. Ghosts, sightings, séances, attempting to reach and speak to the dead, appear very powerfully in Western Culture in the wake of loss on a mass scale. The Civil War in the United States, particularly the South (see Gilpin, 2009), and World War I in Europe, saw an astonishing outbreak in spiritism. Visions of the dead and sightings of religious figures haunted battlefields and post war settings. Freud and Ferenczi were engaged in discussions about the occult and "thought transference," over quite a long period. Their discussions were a mix of fascination, skepticism, and anxiety (see Freud-Ferenczi correspondence, Vol 1; Brabant, Falzeder and Giampieri-Deutsch, 1993; Meszaros, 1994, 2014). We are in the complex domains of unconscious communication. But words like uncanny and haunted are required, the words and language of object relations and internal objects seem too orderly for the experiences the authors in this book are describing.

Despite these cautionary notes, there is the triumph when narrative enters treatment, when fragments and chaos are ordered through naming and genealogy. This has been Davoine and Gaudilliere's (2004) perspective, seeing the long hand of history. It takes a half-century, they felt, to process a war. Unprocessed historical trauma was a prime engine of psychotic functioning. So there is, in the permanent tasks of mourning, both triumph and despair and this must be parsed and held by analyst for the patient and for him/herself.

Consistent with Davoine's thinking, some fifty-plus years after World War II, we are absolutely deluged with memoirs and novels, movies and plays, dances and operas, which are attempting to work through the emotional/psychological aftermath of the Holocaust. Some of these artistic projects have been initiated by second and third-generation survivors in an effort to bear witness to their parents' and grandparents' previously unmetabolized wartime experiences. Some stories take the form of realistic, historically accurate retelling; others are more intuitive and sensory near, like the French film *Le Secret*. In this movie, a boy is born after the war to survivor parents who had lost a son but agreed never to speak about the experience to anyone. Nevertheless, their post-war child is haunted by the spectral presence of his dead brother. Only when his parents finally reveal their loss can their child let go of his brother's ghost, which he had been unconsciously holding for his parents. We wonder if this outpouring of trauma-based artistic endeavors has both a containing and a retraumatizing effect in its conscious effort to put into narrative what is often beyond explaining with words.

We think here of Maya Lin's Vietnam war memorial in Washington DC, with its miles of engraved names of all who were killed. Or the 9/11 memorial in NYC which similarly offers up the engraved names of each of the 2,977 victims on the stone rim surrounding the dramatic multilayered descending memory pools. Perhaps our need for these memorials intensifies as our media-fueled barrage of trauma—absent much space for genuine containment or witnessing—intensifies. In all likelihood, the presence of these memorials does help to counteract absence (Slochower, 2011). But while such public memorials, and the rituals that surround them, are useful, they cannot substitute, says Gaines (1997), for the necessary language and affect accessed through private, internal, personal mourning.

Our attention was drawn both to the wider and larger cultures but also to something closer to home. Ghosts in psychoanalysis, in our profession, our institutes and our theories signify unburied, unmourned losses. In 2014 we read a news story, front page in the New York Times, about the discovery of 55,000 psychiatric patients in unmarked graves in New York. "In New York, more than 55,000 deceased psychiatric patients lie in unmarked graves. Near the former Willard Asylum, a small committee has spent the past three years fighting to memorialize the dead" (Bracken, 2014).

What kind of professional PTSD in our field allowed this to happen, so silently, over a period of so many years? We found ourselves, too, struggling and too often failing to be able to hold on to the specters and fearful shadows that haunt very many psychoanalytic institutes in regard to boundary violations and other moral matters.

The more open we were to looking for ghosts, the more we found them, lurking inside both our patients and ourselves, inside our personal and historical pasts, our internal and external spaces and the architecture of our lives. Ghosts and their ilk (vampires, demons, etc.) are widespread in contemporary popular culture. The television series *Lost,* for example, involves a constant oscillation between fantasy and reality, with none of the containing real-world limits of time and space. People die and reappear and ghosts wander about with an alternating comforting and alarming presence, as they simultaneously revisit their pasts, which are filled with dark secrets and unresolved trauma. Numerous other television series also explore similar experiences of people traumatically gone missing, and the psychological impact on those left behind.

We wonder why contemporary culture seems, right now, particularly strongly pulled toward the world of ghosts, of haunting? Could it be that we are living in a time of greater general uncertainty and chaos in the world—socially, economically—around the globe? Could it be the accumulated mass traumas and losses of modern day warfare, in concert with the fact that these events are no longer reported in a contained way on the 6 o'clock news and in the morning newspaper, but instead broadcast incessantly in excruciating, lurid detail on 24-hour news channels like CNN and across countless portholes on the internet all day and night long? It is harder—for better and worse—to shut out what is going on in the world. But it is also harder to metabolize the abundant and raw exposure.

The internet may play a role in another context. "Ghosting" is a common term in online parlance. It refers to someone (usually within a dating reference) who simply disappears on another person, after extensive online talking or several dates or even months of dating. The use of "ghosting" to describe this commong occurrence indicates a familiarity with the language and experience of ghosts, both more awareness of and literally more ghosts in people's lives. It emphasizes the there/not there of present absences and absent presences of relationships both fostered and maintained online, even post break up. Since this use of the term is also about loss that cannot be processed—because people simply disappear without explanation, because they remain both here—visible online — but not here. These are also absences that haunt.

This book was written with a companion book in mind: *Ghosts in the Consulting Room: Echoes of Trauma in Psychoanalysis.* The two books are distinctly different yet also overlapping. They are enigmatic in their differences, much like the feel of ghosts themselves. We like to think of the two books as mutable: sometimes very distinct, sometimes doppelgängers. A doppelgänger is defined loosely as a ghostly apparition, or alter ego, of a living person. The word originates from the German, literally meaning double-goer or double walker. Further definitions include a ghostly double of a living person that haunts its living counterpart, or a wraith (e.g., astral body or shadow). We want to emphasize the doubleness or existence of the shadow of the other. Much like figure/ground matrices, which can be fluid and shifting, it is often difficult—and intended to be difficult—to tell ghosts and demons apart. What on the surface may seem to be dichotomous categories are actually overlapping in complex, most certainly non-dichotomous ways. Trauma occurs on a continuum. Yet we hope the subtle conceptual distinctions help to illuminate the manner in which one is haunted by ghosts, and demons, distinct and overlapping.

Another of the many potential ways to think of the differences between ghostly present absences and demonic absent presences is to think of the major clinical tasks at hand. In this book and its companion, we are talking about the need to process overwhelming pain and resolve mourning, oftentimes trauma and mourning that have been put off from one generation to another. In *Ghosts in the Consulting Room*, we are trying to address the difficulties and challenges and sometimes limits of mourning. In this book, we are writing about the near-impossibilities of mourning, the stuckness in intractable melancholia (Freud, 1914). Seen through the lens of language, many authors in *Ghosts in the Consulting Room* tend to emphasize verbalization of sorrow and grief, while authors in this book tend to use language having to do with the realm of vampires, dybbuks, demons, and other states of deep and often distorted melancholy, "undeadness" or non-being, elements or substances, organic or inorganic that are not-fully dead, but rather anti-mourning hauntings.

The power of the melancholic state seemed markedly evident to us personally, clinically, and culturally. Most explicitly, we had to notice the tremendous aid that witnessing provides and the alternative difficulties of silence and solitude. This has continued to be part of Gerson's project, tracking the great dangers to witnessing's absence. A great many of our clinical accounts hold absence and silence at the heart of the clinical trauma. Absence and silence are the forms in which ghosts and demons, the wistful, the desparate, and the grotesque may proliferate. Narrative and witnessing are possibly the antidote to haunting. This is the "absence presence that may be created when, as the editors write," There are places and situations and persons and families where knowledge of trauma is refused, where the questions of what happened are turned back unanswered. Perhaps it is there the spirits howl loudest?

*

This is the second of two books on ghosts and demons in twenty-first-century psychoanalysis. It is subtitled: *Echoes of Genocide, Slavery, and Extreme Trauma in Psychoanalytic Practice.*

Working on ghosts and demons required an expansion of vocabulary and imagination. There are ghosts that protect, ghosts that hold us hostage, ghosts that we protect and cannot separate from. But there can be a murderous side to this: demons and vampires, dybuks, and monstrous and grotesque forms that often represent the impossibility of containing and metabolizing loss and trauma. The body and the mind can be the site of attack and invasion. Eros and Thanatos can intermingle and disturb individuals and cultures.

The Consulting Room

Ghosts haunt analyst and analysand, participating in impasses and uncanny experiences in the countertransference and in the transference. While more traditional spiritual practices involving hauntings seek to expel ghosts and demons, psychoanalysis and psychotherapies seek rather to have ghosts readmitted and repatriated.

McGleughlin's chapter, in this book, makes clinical use of haunting photographs by Francesca Woodman to examine excess and unyielding melancholy via ghostly "states of non-being." She makes use of the visual register of Woodman's photographs to help both herself and her severely traumatized patient bring the experience of absence into the workable space of treatment, even without the benefit of conventional language. Atlas' chapter elaborates on how sexual excess can be a conduit for communicating profoundly melancholic ghosts. The author evokes the Hebrew term "the Dybbuk" (defined as a malicious possessing spirit, considered the dislocated soul of a dead person) to help the dyad contain monstrous somatic internalizations. The body is an omnipresent path to accessing nonverbal yet controlling, persecutory spectral presences.

We include Loewald (1960) in this account of the impact of trauma on theory building, wondering what was carried personally for him in the injunction to turn a ghost into an ancestor. Several of our authors draw heavily on him. Kalb elaborates on the Loewaldian notions of ghosts as internalizations gone awry, and then combines it with another originally Loewaldian concept—interpsychic space—to describe how ghosts can come alive in what she calls the "intersomatic" interaction between patient and analyst. Katz uses Loewaldian theory to differentiate "repressed ghosts" from "dissociated vampires" and to explore the emergence of vampires clinically, in what he calls the "enacted dimension" of treatment.

Ghosts remain in various forms and to reprise the insight of Abraham and Torok (1994), in their idea of encrypted identifications, sometimes the secrets passed remain unknown to bearer or receiver. Fox's chapter illustrates how unsettled internalizations and melancholy, in both patient and therapist, can lead to impasse. Fox's account of a fragile and unstable treatment, threatened despite a deep determination in the analyst, opens a difficult possibility for analysts wishing to bear witness. There simply are situations and persons and circumstances in which, despite determination on all sides, mourning may become unbearable even in the holding space of available support, acknowledgment, and witnessing of the consulting room. The therapist is left struggling to metabolize the ghost he is left with when such a patient departs abruptly. It may in retrospect sometimes feel that a patient has arrived in treatment precisely to deposit and leave a ghost, perhaps permanently, perhaps only for a time. The analyst must bear the enigma.

What perhaps most profoundly links all of the chapters in our clinical section is the way that unprocessed gaps, breaches, breaks, opacity, disruptions, cracks, absent presences—actual, fantasized, inherited— lodged in our hearts, bodies, and minds, result in unmetabolized ghosts that haunt our lives and our treatment relationships. It is our human challenge and analytic endeavor to strive to witness, contain, hold, grow from, and try to mourn these ghosts.

Here we think of the release and potential peace of the settling of personal history. But the term also conjures up more collective historical conversations. Here is where Gerson's work is so helpful, his attunement to the potency of contained witnessing, witnessing that allows reflection and linkage, witnessing that is not unduly retraumatizing, witnessing that can facilitate the transformation of present absences and absent presences— whether personally or communally.

The culture and the community

Working on ghosts and demons began for our group in the consulting room but our interests soon burst beyond those confines to the wider world, the world of our institutions and the larger cultures. We have known through many important writers in our field that cultural and social surround leaks into familial and individual experiences (see Aron and Starr, 2012; Corbett, 2009; Davoine and Gaudilliere, 2004; Dimen, 2011; Faimberg, 2004; Puget, 1989; Gentile, 2013).

There are ghosts that haunt our profession, as well. Beginning with our professional father, Freud, we have grappled—and not grappled—with splitting and divisions within our family, boundary violations, and other problematic ghostly present absences and demonic absent presences that live alongside the easier-to-metabolize legacy of meaning-making and the power of the unconscious. In her chapter in this volume, Dimen grapples in a highly personal and evocative way with the damaging absent presence of boundary violations in our field. She discusses her own experience of a violation by her own analyst, and its complicated continuing personal and communal sequelae. It seems clear from her work, and others, that the unprocessed and often unmentionable presence of secret boundary violations perturbs institutional life in our field across all the generations since psychoanalysis' foundation. As we understand more of this matter, it becomes important to see the demonic and vampiric aspects of such secret and unprocessed violations.

The professional history of psychoanalysis was also haunted by the mostly Jewish European psychoanalysts caught in the grasp of WW2. Kuriloff discusses the unspoken and unprocessed effect of their personal histories of persecution and forced immigration on the psychoanalytic traditions that we have inherited. It is striking, in her chapter, to see the ongoing blindspots of analysts and their descendents in their wide-ranging defensive accommodations to the stories of dislocation and phobic hatred.

The preponderance of cultural ghosts is certainly not limited to processing the unthinkably/unspeakably/incomprehensibly enormous losses and consequential haunting of WW2. In his chapter, Etkind writes about the loss of life and hope inherent in the mass deaths of the Gulag, and post-Soviet society's enormous difficulties in beginning to mourn and integrate this "suicide of society." Etkind describes a uniquely Russian cultural form of carnival and the grotesque, which has been tasked with the unbearable process of societal grieving. Also in this volume, Šebek, from Prague, writes of the haunting function of demonic "totalitarian objects"—including the analyst. "Totalitarian objects" are perceived to have "total power;" they stand in as representatives of powerful, cruel ghosts of totalitarian regimes—personal and cultural—from the past. The ghostly uncertainty and emptiness encompassed in such states is explored by Šebek, from clinical and cultural standpoints.

All this inundation with extreme trauma when we have yet to fully acknowledge, bear witness to, and metabolize the grief of our own country's mass traumas of slavery and the devastation of the native American people. Gump writes of the continuing, stultifying haunting among African American descendents of slaves, in a strong voice that needs to be heard. From a place of profoundly painful personal and professional clinical experiences, Gump speaks of the lack of recognition and consequent lack of ability to grieve the enormity of slavery's negation of selfhood.

We circle back to conclude this section of our Introduction with a reprise, a conclusion that resonates deeply with all of our writers. Absence and silence are the forms in which ghosts and demons, the wistful, the desperate, and the grotesque may proliferate. Narrative and witnessing are possibly the antidote to haunting. There are places and situations and persons and families where knowledge of trauma is refused, where the questions of what happened are turned back unanswered. Perhaps it is there the spirits howl loudest?

Note

1 Galit Atlas, Michael Feldman, Heather Ferguson, Arthur Fox, Adrienne Harris, Margery Kalb, and Susan Klebanoff.

Bibliography

Abraham, N. and Torok, M. (1994). *The Shell and the Kernel*. Chicago, IL: University of Chicago Press.

Aron, L. and Starr, K. (2012). *A Psychotherapy for the People; Towards a Progressive Psychoanalysis. Perspectives in Relational Psychoanalysis Book Series*. New York, NY: Routledge.

Baranger, M. and Baranger, W. (2009). *The Work of Confluence: Listening and Interpreting in the Psychoanalytic Field*. London: Karnac Books.

Benjamin, J. (2004). Beyond Doer and Done to: An Intersubjective View of Thirdness. *Psychoanal. Quart.*, 73: 5–46.

Bion, W.R. (1982). *The Long Weekend: 1897–1919 (Part of a Life)*. (Edited by F. Bion). Abingdon: The Fleetwood Press.

Bollas, C. (1994). Aspects of the Erotic Transference. *Psychoanal. Inq.*, 14: 572–590.

Botella, S. and Botella, C. (2005). *The Work of Psychic Figurability: Mental States without Representation*. London: Routledge

Brabant, E., Falzeder, E. and Giampieri-Deutsch, P. (1993). *The Correspondence of Sigmund Freud and Sandor Ferenczi, Vol. 1. 1908-1914*. Cambridge, MA: Harvard University Press.

Bracken, K. (2014). An Asylum's Final Secrets. *New York Times*. Nov 28, 2014.

Caruth, C. (1996). *Unclaimed Experience: Trauma, Narrative, and History*. Baltimore, MD: Johns Hopkins Press.

Casement, P.J. (1982). Samuel Beckett's Relationship to his Mother-Tongue. *Int. Rev. of Psychoanal.*, 9: 35–44.

Corbett, K. (2009). Boyhood Femininity, Gender Identity Disorder, Masculine Presuppositions, and the Anxiety of Regulation. *Psychoanal. Dial.*, 19: 353–370.

Davoine, F. (2007). The Characters of Madness in the Talking Cure. *Psychoanal. Dial.*, 17: 627–638.

Davoine, F. and Gaudilliere, J.M. (2004). *History Beyond Trauma*. London: Other Press.

Deutsch, R. (2014). *Traumatic Ruptures: Abandonment, Betrayal and the Analytic Relationship*. London: Taylor and Francis.

Dimen, M. (Ed.) (2011). *With Culture in Mind; Psychoanalytic Stories*. New York. NY: Routledge.

Durban, J. (2011). Shadows, Ghosts, and Chimaeras: On Some Early Modes of Handling Psycho-Genetic Heritage. *Int. J. Psycho-Anal.,* 92: 903–924.
Faimberg, H. (2004). *Telescoping of Generations.* London: Karnac.
Fraiberg, S. (with Adelson, E., and Shapiro, V.) (1975/1987). Ghosts in the Nursery: A Psychoanalytic Approach to the Problems of Impaired Infant-Mother Relations. In: Louis Fraiberg (Ed.), (1987). *Selected writings of Selma Fraiberg.* Columbus, OH: Ohio State Press, pp. 100–136.
Freud, S. (1909). Analysis of a Phobia in a Five-Year-Old Boy. *S.E.,* X, pp. 1–150. London: Hogarth Press.
Freud, S. (1915). Mourning and Melancholia. *S.E.* XIV. London: Hogarth Press.
Freud, S. (1929). Letter from Sigmund Freud to Ludwig Binswanger, April 11, 1929. *Letters of Sigmund Freud 18731939.* London: The Hogarth Press. p. 386.
Gaines, R. (1997). Detachment and Continuity. *Contemp. Psychoanal.,* 33: 549-571.
Gampel, Y. (1992) Psychoanalysis, ethics and actualities. *Psychoanal. Inq.,* 12: 526–550.
Gentile, K. (2013). Bearing the Cultural in Order to Engage in a Process of Witnessing. *Psychoanal. Psychol.,* 30: 456–470.
Gerson, S. (2009). When the Third is Dead: Memory, Mourning and Witnessing in the Aftermath of the Holocaust. *Int. J of Psycho-Anal.,* 90: 1341–1357.
Gilpin, D.F. (2009). *The Republic of Suffering: Death and the American Civil War.* New York, NY: Vintage.
Goldberg, P. (2008). Catastrophic Change, Communal Dreaming and the Counter-Catastrophic Personality. Paper read at 4th EBOR Conference, Seattle, WA. Nov 1, 2008.
Grand, S. (2010). *The Hero in the Mirror: From Fear to Fortitude.* New York. NY: Routledge.
Grotstein, J. (1998). Review of W.R. Bion, War Memoirs, 1917–1918. *J. of Analytic Psych.,* 43: 610–613.
Harris, A. (2005). Conflict in Relational Treatment. *Psychoanal. Quart.,* 74: 267–293.
Harris, A. (2009). You must Remember This. *Psychoanal. Dial.,* 19: 2–21.
Harris, A. (2013). Time: Stopped, Started, Frozen, Thawed. *The Candidate.* 3: 59–61.
Harris, A. and Sinsheimer, K. (2008). The Analyst's Vulnerability: Finetuning and Preserving Analytic Bodies. In: F. Anderson (Ed.) *Bodies in Treatment.* New York, NY: Routledge.
Laub, D. (2005). Traumatic Shutdown of Narrative and Symbolization: A Death Instinct Derivative? *Contemp. Psychoanal.,* 41: 307–326.
Levine, H., Reed, G. and Scarfone, D. (2013). *Unrepresented States and the Construction of Meaning: Clinical and Theoretical Contributions.* London: Karnac.
Loewald, H. (1960). On the Therapeutic Action of Psychoanalysis. In: *Papers on Psychoanalysis,* 221–256. Maryland, MD: University Publishing Group, Inc.
Loewald, H. (1989). *Papers on Psychoanalysis.* New Haven, CT: Yale University Press.
Meszaros, J. (2014). *Ferenczi and Beyond: Exile of the Budapest School: Solidarity in the Psychoanalytic Movement in the Nazi Years.* London: Karnac.
Ogden, T. (1992). The Dialectically Constituted/decentered Subject of Psychoanalysis. *Int. J. of Psycho-Anal.,* 73: 517–526.
Puget, J. (1989). Social Violence and Psychoanalysis in the Argentinian Context. *Brit. J. Psychother.,* 5: 363–369.
Puget, J. (2002). The State of Threat and Psychoanalysis: From the Uncanny that Structures to the Uncanny that Alienates. *Free Associations,* 9: 611–648.

Reis, B. (2011). Zombie States: Reconsidering the Relationship Between Life and Death Instincts. *Psychoanal. Quart.,* 80: 269–286.
Rozmarin, E. (2011). To Be Is to Betray: On the Place of Collective History and Freedom in Psychoanalysis. *Psychoanal. Dial.,* 21: 320–345.
Slochower, J. (2011). Out of the Analytic Shadow: On the Dynamics of Commemorative Ritual. *Psychoanal. Dial.,* 21: 676–690.
Stern, D. (2015). *Relational Freedom: Emergent Properties in the Relational Field.* London: Routledge.

Clinical

Chapter 1

Ghosts in the consulting room
Reluctant ancestors

Margery Kalb

Ghosts are internalizations gone awry. They arise unbidden, haunting patient and analyst alike—absent presences within us, materializing in the form of repetitive, painful (re)enactments. In this way, ghosts of the past take possession of the present, resisting being "laid to rest as ancestors" (Loewald, 1960). Ghosts are thus reluctant ancestors.

Charlie's ghosts are conspicuous by way of their amorphous, seemingly absent, presence. Nearly 13 years into Charlie's analysis I still know startlingly little about the impaired internalizations that haunt him. And a great deal. For despite the manifest ambiguities of a patient's verbal history, ghosts are insistently undead (Abraham & Torok, 1975/1994; Fraiberg, 1975/1987; Freud, 1909, 1917; Gerson, 2010; Green, 1986/2005; Loewald, 1960). Old, unwelcome ghosts that we try to quash into the cracks and crevices slip out to terrorize Charlie and me, lodging in the somatic "enacted dimension" of the treatment relationship (Katz, 2014). Disavowed phantom presences gather in the shadows to renew their energy and reemerge—violently commandeering our attention to make their poisonous presence acutely felt.

In the earliest years of treatment, especially, I grew physically ill sitting with Charlie. I would break out into a panicky sweat, feeling slightly queasy and very dizzy—barely able to breathe, much less focus on his words. Sessions were eerie and oppressive, teeming with fear; I felt helpless in the face of a virtually unbearable "nameless dread" (Bion, 1962, 1965/2002).

Charlie, then in his late 30s—obese and very dark and intense—spoke with little emotion and in only the most nebulous terms about an unremittingly horrific childhood and a not-much-better present. He described a history riddled with brutal victimization (rapes and physical abuses) from early childhood straight through to adulthood, as well as addiction, self mutilation, run-ins with authority, miserably failed careers and relationships and psychiatric hospitalizations. The picture he painted was relentlessly bleak, and blurry in its details. A rare point of clarity and continuity was Charlie's fear and dread; although the origins and objects of his fears were murky and inconsistent, the panicky feeling itself was tangible, omnipresent, and regularly articulated—Charlie's own nameless dreads.[1] In perpetual flight, Charlie had lived a peripatetic existence in places too numerous to count, with each geographic location representing a different "persona." He was fascinated with dying—not with being dead, but with dying. He spoke disturbingly of his enthrallment with the rotting insides of bodies, and wrote poetry replete with concrete graphic details of freshly decaying near-corpses. Charlie felt surprised, misunderstood and fearful when others were repelled by his ideas. Indeed, much of Charlie's internal life was a lavish world of preoccupation with physical evil, malignant others, gory decomposition. Contradictions abounded, too: even his age, cultural heritage and sexual orientation were equivocal. Specifics of his childhood trauma were murkier still, "memories" changing though remaining equally opaque, over time. And despite his cautiously unobtrusive, meet, and exceptionally obsequious manner, that resulted in my unsettling sense that he was slipping in and out of the room like a shadow, Charlie paradoxically spoke about his insistent dread of others being "mad"—not angry but "mad"—at him. Not coincidentally, parental "madness"—also mostly undefined—was an ongoing touchstone for Charlie. Mirroring his fear of others' madness, he also spoke, softly, scarily (but abstractly), of being evil and of his power to hurt others. Charlie's presence felt aggressively absent to me, as thin as poison air that can suffocate.

I consulted with a colleague and confided that in our joint fear of the enraged pain of his "psychotic core" (Eigen, 1977; Green, 1986/2005; Klein, 1948; Loewald, 1979a, 1979b) I did not see how I could possibly help Charlie and that I wanted to refer him to another therapist. I was urged to contain and continue. Cumulatively and over time, the fearsome unmetabolized affect in the room became overpowering. One day, I stood up at the end of a typically nightmarish, nameless dread-filled session with Charlie—simply stood up—and felt a sudden migraine-like pain behind my eyes, followed by excruciating dizziness. I yelped involuntarily, but single-mindedly managed to get Charlie out the door. And then, I fainted.

As we began the next session, Charlie, predictably, said, "You know, when you yelped, I thought I did that to you. Because I'm too toxic for anyone who comes into contact with me." Charlie has many times asserted that one of us must die. Two people cannot survive and thrive in relationship. Like vampires, one person must be "sucked of vitality" so that the other may live—or, more accurately, remain undead.[2] "If I do better, if you help me do better, you'll get contaminated, sick or something, and it'll be my fault." Under these conditions, "How dare I?" became Charlie's frequent refrain: how dare I enjoy, flourish, desire, love; how dare I live? Inhabited by ghosts, one *becomes* a ghost. Paradoxically, despite my manifestly unwelcoming (Ferenczi, 1929) feelings toward Charlie and his undeadness—which I presume repeats an aspect of Ferenczian unwelcomeness in his early childhood—my psyche, through my body, was/is permeable and receptive to the imploding ghostly visitations emanating from his psyche. Thus are the traumatic ghosts embodied and made available in the potential goldmine and landmine of our "interpsychic" (Bolognini, 2011; Loewald, 1970, 1979)[3] space: in his material bodily preoccupations and thin-as-poison-air destructiveness, and my illness and fainting.

The session at the conclusion of which I fainted was a typically intense one. Consultation with colleagues detected nothing out of the ordinary or explanatory in the manifest verbal content of the session. One theme of his rather confusing stories was how hard it was for Charlie to interact with authority figures and get help: "they" would blame Charlie, calling him "mad" or "crazy." In his customary deadpan monotone, Charlie continued, speaking about how it is his "fault," because he "let a crazy person in" and how much he feared going anywhere, "because I thought they knew, that they talked about it. I feel like a sleaze surrounded by innocents, and I'll contaminate them . . . And everyone can see it, unless I hide my own body, or stay fat. Or stink. I shouldn't be involved with anyone. They're pure and innocent, I'm tainted." After minimizing my anemic attempt to recognize some similar themes in our relationship, Charlie concluded the session in his characteristically obfuscating and mostly affectless way, by recounting experiences of childhood sexual molestation and severe parental "punishment," as well as his associated tendency to avoid or run from relationships.

Intense material? Certainly. But verbally, this was a standard working session, for us. My illness, my paranoia, my nameless dread—though too disruptive for me to track precisely during the course of the session—also began very early in the hour and vacillated, as usual, throughout. And despite the obvious transference-countertransference parallel just beneath the surface of Charlie's words, the dynamic—and the emotion it held—was, typically, mostly throttled: verbally unrecognizable and unmobilizable. It was like being buried alive in a crypt. Together. Even when I occasionally could formulate words, they usually backfired. Words were extremely frightening to Charlie. I was not aware of anything new or different in this session. My fainting took me by surprise. Fear and dread of madness and mortal danger—his/mine/ours—seemed to settle into the body. Had Charlie's toxic ghosts contaminated me? Was I an "innocent" being asphyxiated—bitten and buried alive—by his "taintedness?" Who are these ghosts, exactly? How much were they Charlie's personal ghosts and how much were they the unformulated or unconscious ghosts of his parents' histories? How were we tapping into my personal ghosts? I was mystified.

Indeed, the utter evacuation of feelings and meanings—as was true in Charlie's speech—annuls words, destroying the potential for symbolization and synthesis that might eventually help us lay ghosts to rest. The words of our clinical process were exceptionally opaque. Charlie's narrative, too—his personal, brutally traumatic experience, as well as what was transmitted transgenerationally—was shadowy and verbally obscure. Narrative information about Charlie's ghosts was insubstantial, mysterious, uncanny, unsettling. Toxic air. Without a more articulated history and clinical process, these ghosts were very opaque. Yet this opacity is in keeping with what makes ghosts ghosts. By definition, ghosts are presences that elude yet intrude, to haunt and frighten us. They cannot yet be put into words. During sessions, there was a terror-driven disconnect between the actual verbal content of sessions and what was transpiring beneath the words. The inchoate, absent presences of Charlie's history thus haunt by contagion, emerging enigmatically in mostly nonverbal form—which makes this chapter a peculiar and fraught proposition: How to use mere words to describe the unspeakable? The vagueness of some aspects of this chapter thus replicates the vagueness of Charlie's history, as well as the vagueness between us in the consulting room. The gaps and absences in language reflect the gaps and absences within. In the face of this dearth of explicated events and experiences, the reader may feel nearly as mystified and disequilibriated as I felt in the consulting room, on this dizzying journey into what I will be calling "interpsychic-intersomatic" territory.

The poison air that enveloped Charlie and me left me feeling utterly helpless, gagged, and suffocated. Were these aspects of the unmetabolized ghosts? The atmosphere between us remained petrified until, a few months after I fainted, Charlie came up with his own solution. Charlie took flight—both to protect us and to kill us off—in the form of attending graduate school overseas. I felt relieved, yet also wondered if this was his way of titrating the intensity of the sessions and continuing treatment? I tried to "survive" by offering Skype sessions—and he helped me/us to survive by taking me up on my offer.

In retrospect, although the seven years of Skype sessions seem to have been, as Harris (2009) might call it, an extended "impasse in mourning," they also seemed to serve as a safe-enough bridge: The computer as disembodied Third. Relatively solid ground. My acute physical symptoms subsided. Deeper, in-person engagement (with self and other) and mourning were temporarily suspended and replaced by a more tolerable connection at a safer distance that allowed us a space in which to work together. Via computer, we held each other close, and kept one another at bay, neither fully present nor fully absent.

Not surprisingly, Charlie spent much of his time in school feeling horrifically persecuted and abused by the faculty: "they" who were "mad" at Charlie, and "trying to get rid" of him. In sessions, we frequently pondered his many crises and clashes with authorities and linked these to his history, and his fears of graduating, and his trepidation about what might emerge in our relationship were he to return to NY. To say that the deepest essence of Charlie's treatment is nonverbal is not to say that words, and insight, were never helpful. For example, our Skype sessions spent processing his persecutory anxieties (and linking them to his history) helped Charlie to contain his formidable impulses to run from school. Words—particularly at the safer and more balanced distance of Skype—helped. Yet while words have multiple effects in any treatment, in this one so very little could be articulated, so much was mystifyingly overwhelming, and what could be voiced was so inadequate to touch the deepest levels of Charlie's intrapsychic self.

Supported by his intellectual talents as well as by our Skype sessions, Charlie persevered and surprised himself—"How dare I?"—by graduating. He then surprised both of us—"How dare I?"—by managing to return to NY, to continue sessions in-person. And, perhaps unsurprisingly, that's when all hell broke loose between us. More about that, later.

"Ghosts": An explanation

Ghosts, vampires and related phenomena (Zombies, Doppelgängers, Dybbuks, Draugrs, etc.) have proliferated historically—elusive but compelling presences, as revealed by their abundance in art, photography, film, television, campfire stories, fairytales, literature, ballet, opera and séances, to name just a few. *The Epic of Gilgamesh,* a Sumerian poem that some say is the oldest known work of literature, has dead people stalking the living and eating them. What all these less-than-human, less-than-fully-alive creatures share, is their lack of humanity and aliveness. One wonders whether the sociocultural preoccupation, through the ages, with ghosts and their ilk reflect their ubiquity in our psychic midst, including our struggle to cultivate our humanity and feel more fully alive. Freud (1909) noted almost in passing that "a thing which has not been understood inevitably reappears; like an unlaid ghost it cannot rest until the mystery has been solved and the spell broken" (p. 122). In 1919, Freud defined the uncanny as, "that class of the frightening which leads back to what is known of old and long familiar" (p. 220). Loewald (1960) expanded upon Freud's ideas, in the oft-quoted and evocative, emotional soul of his article "On the Therapeutic Action of Psychoanalysis":

> The transference . . . is due to the blood of recognition, which the patient's unconscious is given to taste so that the old ghosts may reawaken to life. Those who know ghosts tell us that they long to be released from their ghost life and led to rest as ancestors. As ancestors they live forth in the present generation, while as ghosts they are compelled to haunt the present generation with their shadow life. Transference is pathological insofar as the unconscious is a crowd of ghosts. . . .ghosts of the unconscious, imprisoned by defenses but haunting the patient in the dark of his defenses and symptoms, are allowed to taste blood, are let loose. In the daylight of analysis the ghosts of the unconscious are laid to rest as ancestors whose power is taken over and transformed into the new intensity of present life, of the secondary process and contemporary objects.
>
> (pp. 248–249)

Loewald's topographic (conscious vs unconscious/repressed, light vs dark) leanings are simultaneously imbued with multifaceted structural and developmental shadings: He speaks beautifully, in this paper and elsewhere (1962, 1973, 1979a, 1979b), of the interplay between the unconscious and the preconscious, of potential organization and synthesis at relatively higher levels, of a free exchange between mutually influencing systems, of a regressive and progressive, fluid back and forth flow of growth where organization first requires disorganization and conflicts "wane" rather than "resolve." Trained by interpersonalists as well as by Freudians, Loewald epitomizes the potentials of thoughtful integration. And Loewald's language implicitly captures the mystery at the heart of what we do as psychoanalysts: We do not know, really, how one unconscious communicates with another unconscious, how intergenerational transmission of ghosts really works, how interpsychic communication operates; we know only that it does happen—that ghosts haunt.

Ghostly absent presences (re)materialize in the therapeutic relationship, generating nonlinear developmental potential that can unblock pathways for "laying ghosts to rest as ancestors." But Loewald does not give us a clinical map. Resonant as his ideas are—and much as his metaphors of "tasting blood," in the transference-countertransference can be expanded to encompass my clinical experience of psychic vampirism, with Charlie—I have wondered how to find my way along the passageways to the "daylight of analysis." How can we integrate Loewald's ideas into the clinical setting? What enables us to transform ghosts into ancestors? In particular, what facilitates the transformation when the ghost is a vampire whose primary goal is to remain in an undead state, using the analyst's "blood" *not* for "recognition" but rather to sustain undeadness? How can we welcome, let alone tame, noxious internalizations that are obscure and unnamed yet exert a toxic impact on the analyst as well as on the patient, imperiling the therapeutic relationship? Vampires may be an especially intractable kind of ghostly presence, a massively dissociated part of the self that—far more than longing to be laid to rest—wishes to remain unintegrated and hauntingly undead (Katz, personal communication, 2013). But even Loewald's ghosts, who "long to be released from their ghost life," are highly ambivalent in their yearning to be finally buried; ghosts—whether or not in vampire form—are, after all, attachments—adhesive by their very nature. Thus, ghosts are thus reluctant ancestors.

Although Loewald did not publish his "On Internalization" paper until 1973, he was working on it at the same time as he was writing "On the Therapeutic Action of Psychoanalysis," which was published in 1960. It is not a huge leap to imagine that some of the ideas in these articles can be linked, and my explanation of ghosts explicitly connects and extends theory from both articles. In addition, I am highlighting clinical difficulties involved in laying ghosts to rest. In so doing, I am also incorporating a third, later, Loewaldian concept, the clinically salient term "interpsychic" (1970, 1979), into my thinking about ghosts. In thinking about ghosts, I thus link and expand upon these three Loewaldian concepts. I will discuss what I see as the hallmarks of ghosts: underinternalizations (i.e., internalizations that are lacking, inadequately developed or insufficiently usable)[4] involving repression and dissociation; a high degree of compulsive repetition; and undermourned losses; as well as concomitant clinical (re)enactment that emerges by way of interpsychic space.[5]

For me, "ghost" is an umbrella term, a "soft assembly" (Harris, 2008) enfolding the consequences of interacting continuums of personal as well as intergenerationally bequeathed underinternalizations[6] and their sequelae. I think about ghosts as underintegrated, undermetabolized, undersymbolized, underrepresented[7] aspects of early object relationships; they are inchoate, spectral, eerie, undead psychic imprints that colonize body and soul, resulting in highly phenomenologically disturbing states. They are similar to a "shadow of the object" (Freud, 1917), an "unformulated experience" (Stern, 1997), an "unthought known" (Bollas, 1987) that are neither inside nor outside, neither internalized nor uninternalized, neither fully dead nor fully alive, affect saturated yet elusive. For any individual, the degree to which ghosts cast a shadow over a person's life is determined by the extent to which varying continua of underinternalizations, repressions and dissociations dominate; and by the quality, mixture and interrelationships within and amongst these factors. With Charlie, for example, it was impossible to draw constructively on solid-enough internalizations. It is in this sense that ghosts reflect internalizations gone awry. The extreme opacity and undersymbolized nature of Charlie's brutal history, and his wounded internal objects, engendered vampire ghosts that sought nonverbal means of expression; our "knowledge" has been hard-won, erupting mostly in an interpsychic somatic transmission of terrifying, primal bodily transmissions—such as fainting.

With respect to internalizations, there is not simply one ghost. Relationships and their underinternalizations are multiple and overlapping, nestled into one another. Also, object representations are rarely simply "good objects" or "bad objects;" rather, what I call mixed objects (partially "good," partially "bad") proliferate, making the quality of internalizations variable. Consequently, the degree to which any internalized relationship haunts is likely to be mixed and fluid, both because the internal object relationship itself is mixed and because different aspects of that relationship may prevail (or be woven into the tapestry with other object relationships) at different times.[8] For example, at different moments Charlie can speak about aspects of his relationship with his mother quite differently. Mostly, he says things like: "When I was little and I told my mother I was raped she didn't believe me, she was mad. And she'd hit me and lock me in the basement and tell me I'm evil. And I *am* evil. It's all my fault, really. And I think everyone knows, and talks about it . . . " But occasionally, aspects of Charlie's relatively more benign internalizations creep in: "Sometimes my mother can be a little bit nice to me. She let me have a pet. Or loaned me money." Even for Charlie, whose internalizations often seem unremittingly horrific, his mother is a mixed object. These problematic and mixed ghosts appear in the interpsychic space of the analytic interaction, as exemplified by the times I feel like a relatively benevolent mother with Charlie, as well as the times I feel so terribly dizzy and inept.

With respect to repression and dissociation, ghostly phenomena can reflect and be reflected by a return of the repressed, the appearance of a dissociated self-state, or—most often—some combination of both. In the sense Loewald (1960) intended, ghosts are rooted primarily in repression of psychic conflict. In saying that ghosts of the unconscious are "imprisoned by *defenses* . . . " (my italics) Loewald implicitly includes all defenses—including dissociation—in his conceptualization. Nevertheless, in 1960, dissociation was not a focus of psychoanalytic attention, and Loewald does not explicitly refer to it. Ghosts as defined here reflect contemporary thinking on the vital developmental intertwining of both repression and dissociation: Both are disruptive to processes of internalization and integration.[9] Vampires are a subset of ghosts who need to prey on and contaminate in order to remain undead; they arise when more primal forms of dissociation are needed to defend against overwhelming Traumatic experiences and relationships (Katz, personal communication, 2013). With Charlie, the prominence of psychic vampirism and dissociated, somatized Trauma is, for now, very much in the foreground; repression-related ghosts may emerge more robustly later in his analysis. As Smith (2000) cautions, we invariably see a combination of internal and external, capital "T" and small "t" trauma, dissociation and repression, trauma and conflict. Both repression and dissociation are, after all, alternate ways to ward off pain; we use both.

Memories may be more conscious, symbolized ones—what Freedman (personal communication, April 2002), designated "recollections"—or they may be what he characterized as "reminiscences": nonrepresentational, undersymbolized memories that are encoded in emotions and in the body. According to Freedman, reminiscences can be repressed and/or dissociated.[10] Reminiscences impose a perpetual past because a vital present and future are precluded by repetitive reminiscence of that which is undersymboized. Reminiscences are unwitting attempts to conceal painful psychic imprints. But they are attempts that boomerang when the imprints become involuntarily revivified in the form of fresh experience, in an eternally erupting past-as-present (i.e., memory traces that haunt). Repressed and dissociated "reminiscences" are undermetabolized, underinternalized, underintegrated, "memories-in-action" (Busch, 1995, p. 79)—i.e., ghosts.

The less recollected and integrated aspects of internal object relationships are, the more a person will feel haunted by ghosts that can be neither remembered nor forgotten, only painfully, timelessly, compulsively reminisced and (re)enacted. Ghosts and vampires thus live their shadow life in unconscious and preconscious interpsychic space, taking up residence within and between analyst and patient—surprising confusing, and unsettling both members of the dyad; inviting disturbing and uncanny (re)enactments; threatening impasse. Integration of ghosts requires welcoming, or at least tolerating, their deeply unnerving presence—at intrapsychic, interpersonal and interpsychic levels—which can slowly, incrementally, lead to a living through (Fiscalini, 2004) of the profound and painful mourning process required to lay ghosts to rest. A very tall order.

Finally, ghosts—and their subset, vampires—are also attempts to preserve the connection to the object and to evade separation as well as its attendant grieving. Thus, another essential aspect of ghosts is their relationship to loss. While there is universal resistance to mourning, ghosts—and particularly vampires—imply a heightened struggle against loss and grieving. When Loewald referred to the "shadow life" of ghosts, he was perhaps linking, implicitly, these spectral presences with Freud's (1917) idea that the "shadow of the object fell upon the ego." Loewald's ghosts are, as I see it, an extension of Freud's ideas about melancholia: The ego is haunted by underinternalized phenomena that it can neither mourn and give up nor adequately integrate. And, according to Bergmann (2009), the shadow of the object fallen upon the ego precludes love: If one is unable to separate, mourn, and integrate one is unable to love. In my view, ghosts necessarily entail disrupted mourning—a form of Freud's melancholia.[11] Mourning is a developmental achievement. But mourning is never complete or entirely resolved and ghosts are never fully ancestral; healthy mourning involves both "detachment and continuity" (Gaines, 1997). It is the degree of unmournedness and its fixedness that helps determine the degree of hauntedness, and the capacity for love. In treatment, ghosts revivified provide a potential *nachtraglikeit* (Freud, 1895) a particularly powerful (re)enactment that can be used to rework and foster mourning. But Charlie and I are still living mostly in melancholic, suspended time in the transference-countertransference. His vampire preoccupation is with dying and remaining *un*dead—not with death and the mourning that death can bring. A vampiric shadow of the object continues to haunt Charlie's ego.

Trauma and desymbolized somatic ghosts

Trauma[12] (capital "T") poses its own particular transference-countertransference challenges. Bromberg (1998, 2003) suggests that the path to a patient's dissociated states often emerges via the analyst's internal musings. Ogden (1997) emphasizes the potential of the analyst's reverie, and the rich meanings extracted from what he and the patient are experiencing together, over history. Nevertheless, psychoanalysis—with its traditional injunction to delve into the past and remember—would seem to demand a more specific and coherent narrative than has been generated for Charlie's abusive history and mistrustful, disorganized attachment. If the case of Charlie seems unusually ambiguous or perplexing, it is because it *is*, in fact, both of these things, to us in the consulting room. Again, with Charlie, words are confusing and contradictory, but the experience of traumatic "nameless dread" in the room is vivid and takes over. How can it be that, in the course of treatment, unsymbolized vagueness and titration of affect—running parallel to the narrative, symbolized realm—sometimes promotes growth (Bach, 1985, 2006; Bolognini, 2011; Rosenblum, 2009; Slochower, 2013)? What is the role of witnessing and verbalization in the face of unendurable pain (Gerson, 2010; Reis, 2009)?

Rosenblum (2009) specifically writes of the dangers—for survivors—of speaking aloud about trauma, including the risk of psychotic episodes or even suicide. In the face of "soul murder" (Shengold, 2000), Charlie's verbal opacity and undeadness has paradoxically been essential to his literal survival. The spoken revelation (even the possibility of revelation) of traumatic ghosts can be utterly cataclysmic and devastating: Instead of soothing dread and dangers, verbal meaning can aggravate it, shattering vital defenses against madness, violence, and "How dare I?" feelings.

Clinically, I think the idea of neutrality as an unobtrusive, evenly hovering attention that carries a goal of deep and ongoing respect for nonimpingement and presubjective experience can be particularly helpful with certain traumatized patients: Rather than focusing explicitly on a verbal account of traumatic history (which may be dissociated and/or preverbal, as well as excessively threatening), we can wait, try to hold and contain—giving a patient precious space and seeing what unfolds in the immediacy of the transference-countertransference. We can respect the patient's "area of omnipotence" (Winnicott, 1960, 1965). Words can be used perversely, to subvert or destroy meaning, as much as to convey and create it. And witnessing, an emotional engagement[13] with the unbearable experience of an other, need not necessarily be recognized, contained or metabolized verbally. Indeed, Charlie's insistent vagueness does not give me much choice: My mind goes numb and my body absorbs the fear and violence, containing what it can and giving me valuable affective information when it is overwhelmed. Bach (1985) has written about how "uncanny" affects—or somatizations—can reveal and conceal bewildering preverbal states. Listening to my body can sometimes tell me more than listening to Charlie's words.[14] Bion (1962) counseled us to be a welcoming object capable of receiving the patient's nonverbal projections. But Bion also wrote of "nameless dread," implicitly recognizing that there are limits to what we can welcome, witness, contain and metabolize. Affect, mostly in my body, is often my only clue to that which cannot be spoken. We are pressed into a somatic encounter because words threaten the unbearable.

And so, somatization of ghosts prevails—because, as Freud (1923) famously said, the first ego is a body ego; because our bodies receive and express unconscious, preconscious, dissociated, repressed, mysteriously intergenerationally transmitted emotions, that cannot be contained or metabolized; because underintegrated, undermetabolized, undersymbolized, underrepresented, underinternalized psychic phenomena are timelessly trapped in unformulated, unthought bodily form; because so much of what is inside Charlie is simply, madly, unbearable and undead.

How do I "know" this? Bodies bond. Bodies speak. Sometimes stronger and louder than words. The spectral bond between Charlie and me is ineffable, mostly not in words and very difficult to put any words to. Yet it is possible to have undersymbolized but profoundly meaningful—body ego to body ego—communications about the unbearably raw fear, pain and loss that is undead in the heart of one's heart. "Knowledge" can be clearly communicated in body language—though, as previously noted, such communication makes it very difficult to capture and express how what is "known" is known, in words.

I've noted Charlie's obesity, which he describes as the consequence of trying to swallow emotion,[15] particularly rageful madness, as well as a padding that offers a protective trifecta: Something to hide behind, numbness and security. I've noted his confusion about his physical sexual identity, such that—despite the abundant vampire metaphors (contaminating, biting, fainting, etc.) that could be construed erotically—Charlie has felt like everything and nothing, sexually; what sexuality has been present in the clinical encounter has been largely a kind of libidinal desire imbued with merger longings, which I see as a Kleinian, preoedipal sexuality, or a primarily maternal erotic transference-countertransference such as Wrye and Welles (1998) describe. I've noted Charlie's disturbing preoccupation with rotting parts of the insides of dying bodies. And I've noted his active, paradoxically absent yet threatening physical presence. Charlie's early childhood beatings and rapes, as well as later self-mutilations, are brutally physical and emotional, experiences: An imprint for a bodily language of emotional expression. Though the details of his—and his parents'—repetitive abuses remain murky, Charlie has voiced feeling "petrified." Petrification is preservation, an alternate form of memory, if you will, as revealed in the timeless (Harris, 2009; Stolorow, 2003), vampire-like undeadness that haunts Charlie—and the terrible helpless rage, pain and need pulsating just beneath the petrified surface.

(Re)Enactment as yours, mine and ours: interpsychic-intersomatic transmission of ghosts

Embodiment of emotion brings us to what Katz (2011, 2014) refers to as the ongoing, enacted dimension of the relationship between Charlie and me—the space where trauma finds it haunting ground. Katz defines the enacted dimension as the *continuous*, interpsychically created aspect of all treatment relationships. This dimension evolves, unconsciously, side by side with and woven into the more verbally symbolized dimension of the treatment. In the enacted dimension, the analyst—without intent—plays a role in actualizing the patient's unconscious object relationships and traumatic experience. Enacted experience will crystallize around and activate something real in the intrapsychic makeup of the analyst, as well. What our minds cannot or will not recognize enters the more receptive interpsychic space, where most transference-countertransference (re)enactment takes place. The interpsychic is a realm rife with undersymbolized emotions and somatizations, where "reminiscences" reign and the somatic transmission of ghosts flourishes.

Although Freud's early interest in hysteria, trauma and the body ebbed while psychoanalysis turned more to other areas of interest, the body as an essential dimension of the psyche was originally and quintessentially a Freudian notion. Recently, across orientations, there has been renewed psychoanalytic interest in the body—not only as the site of emotional expression, but also as the medium for interpersonal somatic transmission. In particular, there is a burgeoning contemporary literature on interpersonal/relational aspects of somatization. For example, Vartzopoulos and Beratis (2012) recently wrote: "the body demonstrates the vicissitudes of a disorganizing object's presence" (p. 658)" Ferro (2003) described his countertransference headache with a patient as a harbinger of emotion, a material, physical "living" of overwhelming feelings that precedes speaking about them. Following their description of an interaction with a patient who felt dizzy in session, the Barangers (2008) stated:

> The participation of the body in the analytic situation is by no means limited to the patient. Every analyst participates in the physical ambiguity and responds with his or her own body to the patient's unconscious communication.... we could call this phenomenon 'corporeal projective counteridentification.' In these bodily manifestations the analyst responds to an invasion by the patient ... as if the analyst had taken on a physical reaction that the patient should be feeling.
>
> (p. 802)

Grand (2010) wrote of the analyst choosing "transfiguration," by entering into, "alien forms" and allowing oneself to be informed by the richness of our fears and our bodies. She sees the analyst's body as an opening for feared experience, beyond what is verbally explicable. Grand also points out that our cultural vernacular expression of strength, "You can't take this lying down," can shore up the omnipotent rescue fantasies of our therapist self. My therapist self is certainly felled when I feel faint, going limp and vulnerable in bodily recognition of overwhelming, unspoken, confusing and underprocessed aggressive affect.

From their unique perspectives, each of these writers is noticing strong and unusual, mysterious, reactions in the analyst that express a communication between patient and analyst. I would like to link such enactment and somatization with what I am calling the interpsychic-intersomatic transmission of ghosts, by which I mean body ego to body ego transmission via the interpsychic register. Despite our frequent resistance to listening to it, the body is the site of much knowledge. The literal—and often eerie—embodiment of unspeakable traumatic affect, for both of us in Charlie's analysis, reflects our limits in metabolizing, symbolizing and integrating ghastly, ghostly horror. The patient's body is a container for trauma and madness; the analyst's body, in interpsychic space, becomes mobilized as a vicarious container for unconscious and dissociated parts of the self, nameless dreads that the patient cannot tolerate. As a container, the body leads Charlie and me into the unknown, primordial territory that lies outside of immediate shared reflectivity. The stunning opacity of his history is matched by the stunning communication in the psyche-soma sphere—by way of interpsychic-intersomatic transmission. If I can witness and survive the vicarious traumatization, my bodily experience may provide an opportunity to reconstitute the unbearable and reorganize (under)internalizations. It is through the inchoate, malignant affect felt in my body, that we have come to understand and name the "creepy" parts of Charlie—such as his deep identification with madness, with the aggressor, and his murderous rage—which he and I so dread. My illness and dizziness—a literal physical dysregulation and destabilization—is thus a visceral connection to (an identification with) his madness and his fractured, traumatized self—as well as my resistance to those states. My heightened internal orientation and self observation during sessions with Charlie emerge partly from feeling too ill to fully engage or focus on his words; communication is enacted more at the interpsychic-intersomatic than at the interpersonal level.[16]

Dovetailing with Loewald's (1960, 1973a, 1973b, 1976, 1979a, 1979b) emphasis on the disorganization required for organization and the regression necessary for progression, Bollas (1983) highlights the "capacity for generative countertransference regression." He goes on to describe how:

> ... Each analyst working with, rather than against, the countertransference must be prepared, on occasion, to become rather *situationally ill*, in so far as his receptivity to the reliving of the patient's transference will inevitably mean that the patient's representation of

disturbed bits of the mother, or the father, or elements of the infant self, will be utilized in the transference ... In another area of myself, however, I am constantly there as an analyst, observing, assessing, and holding that part of me that is *necessarily ill.*

(pp. 5–6; italics added)

Although Bollas is not specifically referring to physical illness or to interpsychic space, his thoughts about inchoate but affectively unbearable aspects of a patient's psyche that infect and infuse the analyst imply a logical extension: That is, the possibility of enacted somatization and of interpsychic-intersomatic transfer of disturbing states.

So whose somatization is it, anyway? With Charlie, my physical reaction reflects a fluid who's who of questions permeating our interaction: Who is terrified? Who is filled with "nameless dread?" Who is ill? Who is mad? Who is in danger? Who is a murderer? Who is murdered? Whose ghosts are these? What is yours? Mine? Ours? If, in reading this chapter, one learns nearly as much about the analyst as one does about Charlie, it is because so much of what is "known" about Charlie was communicated via interpsychic-intersomatic transmission, not via narrative. No transference-countertransference is entirely induced or entirely personal; the induced and the personal always blend. Somatization has become a pivotal pathway of the enacted dimension between Charlie and me partly because we both—in our different ways—share a physical sensibility.

My physical self has always been prominent: As a child, I so much loved to run and climb and bike, but also appreciated the feel of bodily stillness and peace while reading a good book. After college, I discovered dance and fell in love with the space it offered—along with music, another visceral experience—to simultaneously lose and find myself in it, expressing something of my internal life physically. And fainting, as a way to escape when there is no other escape, a self-preservative psychic flight as well as a literal embodiment of destruction, unconsciousness and undeadness,[17] has also been an aspect of my physical-psychic landscape. For example: in seventh grade, when viewing a graphic film of a childbirth—and feeling prohibited from leaving the classroom—I passed out. What is essential here is that the physical register is a "home" for both Charlie and me—a home that creates receptivity in me to his unconscious/dissociated choreography, space for me to feel "situationally ill."

Despite my own contribution to the specifics of what we enact, I can count on one hand the number of times in my life that I have fainted; it is a desperate measure that I have never felt any inclination to resort to with any other patient. Did I experience, viscerally, some of the states that Charlie cannot allow himself to feel? To paraphrase Loewald, the patient's ghost (or vampire) tastes the blood of recognition in the analyst's unconscious. In other words, via the interpsychic-intersomatic space of our relationship, there was a breakdown in my capacity to contain and metabolize Charlie's projections such that *Charlie's* unconscious/dissociated, intrapsychic experience became dramatically expressed in *my,* personally receptive, body. The tension in the room was so acute that something had to give. When terrifying affect overwhelms him, Charlie flees cities, people, treatment; barred from leaving a session physically, when affect became more then I could bear, I fainted to flee Charlie and his vampire ghosts. For each of us, the flight is a physical symptom that is both defensive (an attempt to control overwhelming affect) and expressive (of feeling destroyed, collapsed, mad). Feeling undead, as in fainting, is also a connection; a way that I, unwittingly, identify with Charlie's traumatic experience.

We are, Charlie and I, each revisited by our own past in our interaction. My mother's brother died of Leukemia when my mother was about three years old. In addition to losing her brother, my mother temporarily "lost" her mother and father to their mourning. I can vividly recall—40 years after her son's death—the tears welling up in my grandmother's eyes at the mere mention of her son, and how it made me cringe at the heartbreaking depth of her pain. My father's mother died of a sudden virus when my father was just three months old. My parents each experienced something akin to Andre Green's (1986/2005) "dead mother," where a vital, nurturing parent is suddenly and traumatically lost or absent. In unconsciously finding one another and having children, my parents unwittingly passed on a potent legacy of early, unconscious, not-fully-mourned, traumatic loss. And both my parents' losses were due to *physical* illnesses, which links up with my own proclivities toward physicality. Charlie's parents were both, as children, besieged by massive, brutal trauma and loss, which they, in turn, re-inflicted on their children. Helplessness in the face of trauma and loss is a prominent theme for both of us.

Certainly Charlie's intergenerational inheritance and mine are very different, too: While my family history is shadowed by traumatic loss, there is no actual human persecutor or sadist; rather it is a legacy of naturally occurring tragedy, loss, and its attendant absence, which allowed for more relatively benevolent internalizations. By way of his capacity to be undead and his strengths, Charlie has sort-of-survived intentional, malevolently-inflicted, violence that was radically toxic. But the cost of Charlie's survival was undeadness.

In what ways does the intermingling of each of our unique, internal object relations, and the interaction of our ghosts, affect our work? Despite our differences, we are, each of us, haunted by early, preverbal loss. We both experienced, from the very beginning of our lives, the undead ghosts that haunted our parents and a legacy of unmourned grief that we were powerless to repair. As a result, we each carry survivor guilt that leads us, to different degrees, to question what seems "too good to be true," to ask: "How dare I?" And so I am, despite my considerable resistance, personally receptive to Charlie's primal communications in interpsychic-intersomatic space.

For a very long time, toxicity in the room, my inner turmoil, and my concerns about Charlie's possible reaction to his impact on me (and others) made it impossible to consider alternatives to self holding and bracketing (Slochower, 1995/2014) my own feelings. I would soothe and ground myself during sessions by massaging the back of my neck or imagining an enlivening interaction. Writing this paper has also served as a way to contain and metabolize the absent but sinister presences boiling over in our midst. I am convinced that, on a preconscious level, Charlie has always known quite a lot about his impact on me. But it is only recently, having become more aware—and ever-so-slightly less terrified—of some the meanings embedded in my reactions to Charlie, that I have been emboldened to dare: To question whether/when/how much to give back to Charlie, how much is say-able, how much rage and pain can be openly felt, what is survive-able.

All hell broke loose

So: I mentioned that all hell broke loose upon Charlie's return to NY. Charlie left me. Three times. His flights were interspersed with fertile periods that included more direct expression of affect—both aggression and need—and more moments of connection and insight. But the difficulties of contact—the interpersonal, intrapsychic and interpsychic intensity of being embodied, together, in-person, coalesced with growing neediness, here-and-now rage, and "How dare I?" feelings over getting good things, to fuel eruptions of backlash and rupture. The vampire ghosts would gather and eventually swarm to have their say, calling Charlie to leave, leave the land of linkages and depressive position potentials, and rejoin them. From Charlie's perspective, what is all-important in the moment is that flight freezes the vampire's power to contaminate and kill.

What did fertility look like in the midst of the tempest? Alongside the emotional squalls, I saw fledgling progress in Charlie's life: a hard-won job, a boss who was not always experienced as persecutory, an attempt to live in a reliable romantic relationship. And I changed, too. I listened with my body and learned to recognize and track Charlie's anger by my dizziness, verbalizing—and not verbalizing—the rage in the room as means of regulation. Thus we began to understand that we can—sometimes, at least—hover at the edge of what is manageable rather than tumbling into the chasm where the storm rages. But the fertility proved difficult for Charlie to bear.

The following dream signaled the imminent resurgence of Charlie's hostile ghosts: "My boss was giving me enough rope to hang myself. A lethal fungus in the office grew and grew and began crawling up my legs and all over me."

Charlie first wondered whether the slow-growing fungus represented murder or suicide. He went on to question whether "the good stuff might all be a trick, like with my mother who's nice to me sometimes, a tiny bit nice to pull me in, and then if I relax: boom! Like rats get intermittent reinforcement and never know what to expect." I interjected: "Like with me, here?" "Yes!" Charlie replied, "It's bad to trust in them and enjoy. Maybe you manipulated me into coming back here, maybe you and my boss are being nice so I'll relax and trust you, and then: boom. And I'm spoiled and poisonous and rotten because I was raped, so if I succeed and take pleasure I'm just a liar anyway. And alone. Being rotten at least I'm with my [sibling] and my parents. When I feel good I'm alone . . . all this transformation lately is scary."

Shortly thereafter, Charlie came in and announced: "I have bad news: my boss is crazy again; he went on the attack and said I'm too expensive and not doing enough work and can't take the time to go to therapy anymore. This is my last session. I need to take a break." Charlie denied that he was running or ruining, denied that the break might be related to feeling mad or needy or threatened, rejected my concerns about his well-being. He simply insisted that I did not understand the "reality" of his situation. He was already gone, and I was speaking to a different "persona;" I could not reach Charlie.

I marvel at his evisceration of meaning; marvel at his sudden blindness and the force of the repetition compulsion; marvel at the power of this process in which we are swept up. Perhaps these breaks are a version of Charlie's flight overseas: an expression of (and compromise between) his ambivalent wish to both protect us and kill us off. Perhaps Charlie needs to try to kill me and see whether or not I can survive. Perhaps I cannot adequately feel my way into the role of Charlie's malignant seducer. Perhaps Charlie is precipitating absence and loss in an attempt to ward off feeling and mourning old absences and losses. Perhaps the good things in Charlie's life—his graduate degree, a new job, developing relationships—feel too daring. Perhaps the more we can welcome, sit with—and survive—hostility, neediness, and the terror of both, the less Charlie will need to try to sever our relationship. Perhaps, too, Charlie needs to know he can come and go as needed. Perhaps, most of all, it is tempting to try to think our way out of just how scary ghosts are and just how much we do not understand.

Certainly, during the breaks Charlie is an un-patient, an absent ghostly presence I hold in mind for a timeless duration.[18] And certainly, these manic flights leave Charlie (re)shattered and me feeling powerless, angry, vulnerable. When Charlie returns from these breaks, he typically speaks of feeling "fragmented" or having a "meltdown" during the break, even of wanting to die. Hearing his pained experience, my anger and helplessness quickly melt into compassion and concern. And so the waning of the immediate rupture ushers in another period of fertile meaning-making that is, in itself, part of the cyclically enacted interaction.

And so it goes. Ghosts (especially vampire ghosts) are not easily—and never entirely—laid to rest. On the clinical level, the therapeutic action of transforming "ghosts" into "ancestors" is more fraught than Loewald's (1960) theoretical outline recognized. Poison, imbibed early on, becomes easily mistaken for nourishment. We love our ghosts. Change means catastrophe.

As Charlie's analyst, I feel I am asking him to live; but for Charlie, to come alive paradoxically means to kill (murder) and to die (suicide), psychically—another "confusion of tongues." Under such conditions, mourning, reparation, laying ghosts to rest—and aliveness itself—becomes preposterous. Undead vampire ghosts are thus powerfully compelling. They wish to possess us, endlessly—to stop time and, in so doing, destroy any possibility of present or future, any possibility of relatedness born of separateness, any possibility of life. And yet, the nascent hope of an enlarged area of vitality has been born. Can it live? Do we dare?

Notes

1 Related, I believe, to nameless dread, Bion (1976/2005) asserted that, "In psychoanalysis, when approaching the unconscious—that is, what we do not know—we, patient and analyst alike, are certain to be disturbed. In every consulting-room, there ought to be two rather frightened people: the patient and the psychoanalyst. If they are not both frightened, one wonders why they are bothering to find out what everyone knows." See page 5 quote for the source of this quote.
2 Interestingly, Charlie's vagueness about his age, and his sense of timelessness, also resemble a vampire-like state.
3 Expanding Freud's (1915) groundbreaking idea that the unconscious of one person can, uncannily, communicate with the unconscious of another without passing through the conscious, Loewald (1970, 1979) defined the "interpsychic" dimension of the patient-analyst relationship as the *unconscious or preconscious* effect and influence on one another. Bolognini (2011) vividly illustrates the essence of interpsychic space with his metaphor of a cat flap – the swinging flap at the bottom of a door that allows a cat to come and go, freely and unobtrusively. The treatment space provides a cat flap, a portal for this *preconscious* interpsychic communication. In other words, the preconscious uses the flap for interpsychic exchange of that which is undersymbolized and undermetabolized.

After Katz (2014), I distinguish interpsychic communication from the term "intersubjectivity," which is defined differently by different authors and often includes *conscious* awareness of communications as well as a capacity to recognize the separate subjectivity of another (Stolorow & Atwood, 1992). Subjective is, after all, the second half of the word intersubjective, implying something that takes place between two subjects. But this is not always the case. According to Bolognini (2011), the interpsychic includes "presubjective" experience. Bollas (2001) has dubbed the term interpsychic, "Freudian intersubjectivity" for its privileging of unconscious and preconscious communication. Loewald's and Bolognini's definitions of interpsychic communications focus on preconscious and unconscious experience, and also encompass "presubjective" experience — making space for both one-person and two-person dimensions of the experience in the analytic relationship.
4 Since I see internalizations as ranging from "good enough" (i.e., adequate for drawing on constructively), to poor (inadequately developed or otherwise insufficiently usable), I use the term underinternalized, rather than the more usual term uninternalized, throughout this chapter. Similarly, I use the terms undermetabolized, undersymbolized, undermourned, and so on to connote and emphasize a *continuum* of robustness and psychic usability for each these concepts.
5 There are many possible ways to conceptualize ghosts (Baranger & Baranger, 2008, 2009; Durban, 2011; Faimberg, 2005; Freud, 1909, 1917; Fraiberg, 1975; Gerson 2010; Green, 1986, 1993; Reis, 2011; Shengold, 2000). I here footnote just a few prominent theoretical examples, but it is beyond the scope of this chapter to explore all the variations.

Bollas (1987, 1996, 2001) might think of ghosts as disruptive, preverbal, "unthought known" material that can be "recalled" in the transference. He writes that, "Behind the ostensibly offending other (whether analyst or someone else) is the intangible ghost of a profound familiar "other" who inhabits the self and becomes indistinguishable from it (1996: p. 9)." Abraham and Torok (1975/1994) have written about a "ghost" or "phantom" as a "gap in the unconscious, an unknown. . . .a gap without a burial place" (p. 140) created partly by intergenerational "repressed" secrets. Stern (1997), rooted in a dissociation model, might think about ghosts in terms of not-yet-reflected-upon "unformulated experience" – a "gap" in Charlie's experienceable knowledge of himself that is partly a legacy from his parents and partly a legacy of his own, lived, traumatic history. Bromberg (2003), also emphasizing dissociation, has similarly written that, "The truth that is held by a dissociated state as an affective memory without a coherent autobiographical memory of its traumatic origin haunts the rest of the self. It remains a ghostly horror . . . " (p.707). Fonagy (2008), integrating structural and relational approaches, might see ghosts as affective repetitions and the inability to regulate them, resulting from attachment (and other) trauma, and concomitant impaired mentalization processes. From Fonagy's perspective, ghosts could be seen as split off unmentalized processes that are reactivated in the analytic dyad. According to Fonagy, " . . . uncontained self states create disorganization within the self and have to be projected out to be regulated. Hence the frequent recourse to projective identification . . . we have referred to these split off parts of the self as the 'alien self' (p. 21)."

6 Definition of the term "internalization" could easily be a paper unto itself. For current purposes, I follow Loewald's (1973) definition of the term. According to him, in a sturdy internalization the object is "destroyed" and assimilated as part of the self; it is an integration and organization for the psyche (rather than a repression or other defensive process that works against organizationand synthesis).

7 Green (1986, 1993) used the concept "unrepresented" to refer to the failure to represent an object internally (i.e., an absence or absent presence). This failure is never pure, I think. Therefore, I use my term "underrepresented" to connote the particular kind of inadequate internalizations that can occur in the face of emotionally traumatizing experience such as absence or "deadness" in primary caregivers. According to Green, one result of an unrepresented object is that the patient's "love is still mortgaged to the dead [i.e., continually dying, undead] mother (p. 156)." Decathexis, delinking and discontinuity proliferate. I include this adaptation of Green's ideas and language here because themes of deadness/undeadness, absent presence, and work in the negative/destructiveness have suffused the transference-countertransference with Charlie.

8 Internalization of a relatively good enough object relationship can result in what some might be tempted to call a "good ghost," but "good ghosts" are unlikely to disturb or wreak havoc in the consulting room; in fact, what might be designated a "good ghost" is more simply thought of as an "ancestor": a good-enough internalization that has become a relatively integrated, metabolized part of the self.

9 Repression and dissociation are distinct terms. I frequently use them together because I see the two processes as embedded in one another. Both develop, and co-exist, in the same person, and both contribute to the creation of underinternalizations and ghosts (and, concomitantly, continual reenacting and living in a petrified past).

Additionally, one consequence of both repression and dissociation is that ghosts may be passed from generation to generation. While Fraiberg's (1975/1987) ghosts are bred of intergenerationally transmitted Trauma with a capital "T" (massively derailing, overwhelming experience with extensive long term sequelae, including severe dissociation), ghosts need not necessarily be the result of capital "T" Trauma. Small "t" trauma (*relatively* less massively derailing, in experience and in long-term consequences) and psychic conflict that eventuate in repression also result in the intergenerational transmission of ghosts. Ghosts emanate from both kinds of trauma, from both repression and dissociation.

Clinically, dissociated ghosts seem to fight harder against symbolization, insight, mourning and being laid to rest as ancestors. Either repression or dissociation tends to be the prominent experience with a certain patient or at a certain time in treatment.

10 Freedman (personal communication, 2002) expanded upon Breuer & Freud's (1893), Freud's (1914), and Loewald's (1953, 1973, 1976) ideas of "reminiscences" to explicitly include dissociated, as well as repressed, experiences and memories. Such an inclusion also led him (Freedman & Russell, 2003) to reject a clinical dichotomy between interpretation and insight, on the one hand, and implicit relational knowing and intersubjective relatedness, on the other, stating that there is no "one path toward

change (p. 82)." This certainly seems borne out, over time, with Charlie: different approaches seem to be more helpful at different times in treatment.
11 Indeed, in addition to underinternalization and compulsive reenactment, another feature that I believe differentiates ghosts from "internalized objects" is that ghosts necessarily entail unmourned (or, more precisely, undermourned) losses and melancholia. Adequate internalization is a pre-condition for mourning. However, unlike Freud's (1917) conception of melancholia via repression, ghosts may also include losses undergrieved due to dissociation.
12 For a fuller discussion of trauma, dissociation, and disorganized attachment see, for example, Bach, 2006; Lachmann & Beebe, 1997; Bromberg, 1998, 2001; Davis & Frawley, 1994; Ferenczi, 1929, 1933; Harris, 1996; Howell, 2005; Hurvich, 2003; Knafo, 2004; Laub & Auerhahn, 1993; Lyons-Ruth, 2003; Stolorow, 2003.
13 The three functions of witnessing are defined, for current purposes, as recognition, containment and metabolization. These functions may, together, provide a partial corrective for the trauma of a "confusion of tongues" (Ferenczi, 1949).
14 Interestingly, with respect to the literal body and its psychic sequelae, Abraham and Torok (1994) wrote that " . . . the mother's constancy is the guarantor of the meaning of words . . . The passage from food to language in the mouth presupposes the successful replacement of the object's presence with the self's cognizance of its absence (p. 128)." In the current conceptualization: If constancy is developmentally sufficient, then we can feel a gap, an absence, loss, by recognizing it, and mourning it; but if the mother's constancy is inadequate, loss cannot be recognized (it is more nebulous and difficult to feel loss of something one never had) and what is taken in is a mostly wordless underinternalization that haunts – and presumably haunts the analyst-patient relationship, as well.
15 Abraham and Torok (1994) discussed how "swallowed and preserved" trauma and the associated "Inexpressible mourning erects a secret tomb inside the subject . . . the loss is buried alive" (pp. 130–131) and "encrypted" in the preconscious. Although Abraham and Torok call this process "preservative repression" it sounds, to contemporary ears, quite similar to the traumatic dissociated feelings "swallowed" by Charlie.
16 Numerous authors who have written about psychosis have touched on similar dynamics of identification and distance in the transference-countertransference (Ogden, 1980, 2007; Searles, 1961, 1976, 1977; Williams, 1998, 2004; and others).
17 Is fainting a vertical split, an extreme dissociation? Or is fainting a horizontal split, an unconsciousness? Group discussions (Galit Atlas, Michael Feldman, Heather Ferguson, Arthur Fox, Adrienne Harris, Susan Klebanoff) suggest that passing out may be either an avoidance of dissociation or an extreme form of it. Either way, my fainting signals that Charlie has "destroyed" (Winnicott, 1969) me, or that I "collapsed" (Green, 1986) due to my identification with the undeadness in him.
18 We absorb so much from our patients. Thus, the ghost that a patient leaves, in leaving treatment – perhaps always but particularly unsettlingly when long-term work is interrupted abruptly – leads to an absent presence and complicated grieving in us.

This chapter first appeared as 'Ghosts in the Consulting Room: Reluctant Ancestors' in *Contemporary Psychoanalysis*, Volume 51, Issue 1, 2015. Reprinted by permission of Taylor & Francis, LLC and the William Alanson White Institute of Psychiatry, Psychoanalysis & Psychology and the William Alanson White Psychoanalytic Society (http://www.wawhite.org/).

Bibliography

Abraham, N. & Torok, M. (1994). *The Shell and the Kernel.* Chicago IL: University of Chicago Press. (Original work published 1975.)

Bach, S. (1985). *Narcissistic States and the Therapeutic Process*. Hillsdale, NJ: Jason Aronson, Inc.
Bach, S. (2006). *Getting from Here to There: Analytic Love, Analytic Process*. Hillsdale, NJ: The Analytic Press.
Baranger, M. & Baranger, W. (2008). The analytic situation as a dynamic field. *International Journal of Psycho-Analysis*, 89: 795–826.
Baranger, M. & Baranger, W. (2009). *The Work of Confluence: Listening and Interpreting in the Psychoanalytic Field*. London: Karnac Books.
Bergmann, M. (2009). The inability to mourn and the inability to love in Shakespeare's *Hamlet*. *Psychoanalytic Quarterly*, 78: 397–423.
Bion, W.R. (1962). *Learning from Experience*. London: Tavistock.
Bion, W.R. (2002). *Transformations: Change from Learning to Growth*. London: Karnac Books. (Original work published 1965.)
Bion, W.R. (2005). *The Tavistock Seminars*. London: Karnac Books. (Original work published 1976.)
Bollas, C. (1983). Expressive uses of the countertransference—Notes to the patient from oneself. *Contemporary Psychoanalysis*, 19:1–33.
Bollas, C. (1987). *The Shadow of the Object: Psychoanalysis of the Unthought Known*. London: Free Association Books.
Bollas, C. (1996). Borderline desire. *International Forum of Psychoanalysis*, 5: 5–9.
Bollas, C. (2001). Freudian intersubjectivity: Commentary on paper by Julie Gerhardt and Annie Sweetnam. *Psychoanalytic Dialogues*, 11: 93–105.
Bolognini, S. (2011). *Secret Passages: The Theory and Technique of Interpsychic Relations*. New York, NY: Routledge.
Breuer, J. & Freud, S. (1893). On the psychical mechanism of hysterical phenomena: Preliminary communication from Studies on Hysteria. *SE*, II: 1–17.
Bromberg, P. (1998). *Standing in the Spaces: Essays on Clinical Process, Trauma, and Dissociation*. Hillsdale, NJ: The Analytic Press.
Bromberg, P. (2001). Treating patients with symptoms – and symptoms with patience: Reflections on shame, dissociation, and eating disorders. *Psychoanalytic Dialogues*, 11: 891–912.
Bromberg, P. (2003). One need not be a house to be haunted: On enactment, dissociation, and the dread of 'not-me' – a case study. *Psychoanalytic Dialogues*, 13: 689–709.
Busch, F. (1995). Do actions speak louder than words? A query into an enigma in analytic theory and technique. *Journal of the American Psychoanalytic Association*, 43: 61–82.
Davis, J. & Frawley, M.G. (1994). *Treating the Adult Survivors of Childhood Sexual Abuse: A Psychoanalytic Perspective*. New York, NY: Basic Books.
Durban, J. (2011). Shadows, ghosts, and chimaeras: On some early modes of handling psycho-genetic heritage. *The International Journal of Psychoanalysis*, 92: 903–924.
Eigen, M. (1977). *The Psychotic Core*. New York, NY: Jason Aronson.
Faimberg, H. (2005). *The Telescoping of Generations: Listening to Narcissistic Links Between Generations*. London: Routledge.
Ferenczi, S. (1929). The unwelcome child and his death-instinct. *International Journal of Psycho-Analysis*, 10: 125–129.
Ferenczi, S. (1933). Confusion of tongues between adults and the child. In: *Final Contributions to the Problems and Methods of Psycho-Analysis*. New York, NY: Basic Books Inc. (1955), pp. 102–107.
Ferenczi, S. (1949). Confusion of tongues between the adults and the child – (The language of tenderness and of passion). *International Journal of Psycho-Analysis*, 30: 225–230.

Ferro, A. (2003). Marcella: The transition from explosive sensoriality to the ability to think. *Psychoanalytic Quarterly*, 72: 183–200.
Fiscalini, J. (2004). *Coparticipant Psychoanalysis.* New York, NY: Columbia University Press.
Fonagy, P. (2008). A genuinely developmental theory of sexual enjoyment and its implications for psychoanalytic technique. *Journal of the American Psychoanalytic Association*, 56: 11–36.
Fraiberg, S. (with Adelson, E., & Shapiro, V.) (1975/1987). Ghosts in the nursery: A psychoanalytic approach to the problems of impaired infant-mother relations. In: L. Fraiberg (Ed.), *Selected writings of Selma Fraiberg* (pp. 100–136), Columbus OH: Ohio State Press. (Original work published in 1975)
Freedman, N. & Russell, J. (2003). Symbolization and the analytic discourse. *Psychoanalysis and Contemporary Thought*, 26: 39–87.
Freud, S. (1895). Studies on hysteria. *SE,* II: 1–335.
Freud, S. (1909). Analysis of a phobia in a five-year-old boy. *SE,* X: 1–150.
Freud, S. (1914). Remembering, repeating, and working-through. *SE,* XII: 145–156.
Freud, S. (1917). Mourning and melancholia, *SE,* XIV: 243–258.
Freud, S. (1919). The uncanny. *SE,* XVII: 217–256.
Freud, S. (1920). Beyond the pleasure principle. *SE,* XVIII: 3–23.
Freud, S. (1923). The ego and the id. *SE,* XIX: 1–66.
Gaines, R. (1997). Detachment and continuity. *Contemporary Psychoanalysis*, 33: 549–571.
Gerson, S. (2010). When the third is dead: Memory, mourning, and witnessing in the aftermath of the Holocaust. *International Journal of Psycho-Analysis,* 90: 1341–1357.
Grand, S. (2010). *The Hero in the Mirror: From Fear to Fortitude.* New York, NY: Routledge.
Green, A. (1999). *The Work of the Negative.* London: Free Association Books.
Green, A. (2005). The dead mother. In A. Green: *On Private Madness.* London: Karnac. (Original work published in 1986.)
Harris, A. (1996). The conceptual power of multiplicity. *Contemporary Psychoanalysis*, 32: 537–552.
Harris, A. (2008). *Gender as Soft Assembly.* London: Routledge.
Harris, A. (2009). You must remember this. *Psychoanalytic Dialogues*, 19: 2–21.
Howell, E.F. (2005). *The Dissociative Mind.* Hillsdale, NJ: The Analytic Press.
Hurvich, M. (2003). The place of annihilation anxieties in psychoanalytic theory, *Journal of the American Psychoanalytic Association*, 51: 579–616.
Katz, G. (2011). Trauma in action: The enacted dimension of analytic process in a third generation holocaust survivor. Discussion of "Secretly attached, secretly separate." In A.B. Druck, C. Ellman, N. Freedman, & A. Thaler (Eds.), *A New Freudian Synthesis: Clinical Process in the Next Generation.* London: Karnac Books, Chapter 11, pp. 239–247
Katz, G. (2014). *The Play Within the Play: The Enacted Dimension of Analytic Process.* London: Routledge.
Klein, M. (1948). *Contributions to Psycho-Analysis.* London: Hogarth Press.
Knafo, D. (Ed.) (2004). *Living with Terror, Working* with *Trauma: A Clinician's Handbook.* NJ: Jason Aronson.
Lachmann, F.M. & Beebe, B. (1997). Trauma, interpretation, and self-state transformations. *Psychoanalysis and Contemporary Thought*, 20: 269–291.
Lasky, R. (Ed.) (2002). *Symbolization and Desymbolization: Essays in Honor of Norbert Freedman.* New York, NY: Other Press.
Laub, D. & Auerhahn, N.C. (1993). Knowing and not knowing massive psychic trauma. *International Journal of Psycho-Anal*ysis, 74: 287–302.

Little, M. (1985). Working with Winnicott Where Psychotic Anxieties Prevail. *Free Association.* 5: 1–19.
Loewald, H.W. (1953). Hypnoid state, repression, abreaction and recollection. In: *Papers on Psychoanalysis,* 33–42, Maryland, MD: University Publishing Group, Inc.
Loewald, H. (1960). On the therapeutic action of psychoanalysis. In: *Papers on Psychoanalysis,* 221–256. Maryland, MD: University Publishing Group, Inc.
Loewald, H. (1962). Internalization, separation, mourning, and the superego. In: *Papers on Psychoanalysis,* 257–276. Maryland, MD: University Publishing Group, Inc.
Loewald, H. (1970). Psychoanalytic theory and the psychoanalytic process. *Psychoanalytic Study of the Child,* 25, 45–68.
Loewald, H. (1973a). On internalization. *International Journal of Psychoanalysis,* 54: 9–17.
Loewald, H. (1973b). Some considerations on repetition and the repetition compulsion. In: *Papers on Psychoanalysis,* 87–101. Maryland, MD: University Publishing Group, Inc.
Loewald, H. (1976). Perspectives on memory. In: *Papers on Psychoanalysis,* 148–173. Maryland, MD: University Publishing Group, Inc.
Loewald, H. (1979a). Reflections on the psychoanalytic process and its therapeutic potential. *Psychoanalytic Study of the Child,* 34: 155–167.
Loewald, H. (1979b). The waning of the Oedipus Complex. In: *Papers on Psychoanalysis,* 384–404. Maryland, MD: University Publishing Group, Inc.
Lyons-Ruth, K. (2003). Dissociation and the parent-infant dialogue: A longitudinal perspective from attachment research. *Journal of the American Psychoanalytic Association,* 51: 883–911.
Ogden, T.H. (1980). On the nature of schizophrenic conflict. *International Journal of Psychoanalysis,* 61: 513–533.
Ogden, T. (1997). Reverie and metaphor: Some thoughts on how I work as a psychoanalyst. *International Journal of Psychoanalysis,* 78: 719–732.
Ogden, T.H. (2007). Reading Harold Searles. *International Journal of Psychoanalysis,* 88: 353–369.
Reis, B. (2009). Performative and enactive features of psychoanalytic witnessing: The Transference as the scene of address. *International Journal of Psychoanalysis,* 90: 1359–1372.
Rosenblum, R. (2009). Postponing trauma: The dangers of telling. *International Journal of Psychoanalysis,* 90: 1319–1340.
Searles, H.F. (1961). Schizophrenic communication. *Psychoanalytic Review,* 48A: 3–50.
Searles, H.F. (1976). Psychoanalytic therapy with schizophrenic patients in a private practice context. *Contemporary Psychoanalysis,* 12: 387–406.
Searles, H.F. (1977). The analyst's participant observation as influenced by the patient's transference. *Contemporary Psychoanalysis,* 13: 367–370.
Shengold, L. (2000). *Soul Murder Revisited: Thoughts about Therapy, Hate, Love, and Memory.* New Haven, CT: Yale University Press.
Slochower, J. (2013). Analytic enclaves and analytic outcome: A clinical mystery. *Psychoanalytic Dialogues,* 23: 243–258.
Slochower, J.A. (1995/2014). *Holding and Psychoanalysis: A Relational Perspective.* 2nd Edition. New York, NY: Routledge.
Smith, H.F. (2000). Conflict: See under dissociation. *Psychoanalytic Dialogues,* 10: 539–550.
Stern, D.B., (1997). *Unformulated Experience: From Dissociation to Imagination in Psychoanalysis.* Hillsdale, NJ: The Analytic Press.
Stolorow, R.D. & Atwood, G.E. (1992). *Contexts of Being.* Hillsdale, NJ: The Analytic Press.

Stolorow, R.D. (2003). Trauma and temporality. *Psychoanalytic Psychology,* 20: 158–161.
Vartzopoulos, I. & Beratis, S. (2012). Bodily manifestations in the psychoanalytic process. *Psychoanalytic Quarterly*, 81 (3): 657–681.
Williams, P. (1998). Psychotic developments in a sexually abused borderline patient. *Psychoanalytic Dialogues*, 8: 459–491.
Williams, P. (2004). Incorporation of an invasive object. *International Journal of Psychoanalysis*, 85: 1333–1348.
Winnicott, D.W. (1960). The theory of the parent-infant relationship. *International Journal of Psycho-Analysis,* 41: 585–595.
Winnicott, D.W. (1965). *The Maturational Processes and the Facilitating Environment: Studies in the Theory of Emotional Development.* The International Psycho-Analytical Library, 64: 1–276. London: The Hogarth Press and the Institute of Psycho-Analysis.
Winnicott, D.W. (1969). *The use of an object* and relating through identification. *International Journal of Psychoanalysis*, 50: 711–716.
Wrye, H.K. & Welles, J.K., (1998). *The Narration of Desire: Erotic Transferences and Countertransferences.* New York, NY: Routledge.

Chapter 2

The Dybbuk

It's me or him

Galit Atlas

"Her name's Leah. I sit and think of her every minute, can't stop. I imagine undressing her. Everywhere, on the floor, on the bed, in my office, on the train to Boston. I kiss her body all over. I whisper to her, 'Leah. I love you. I need you.'" Danny looks at me, smiling sadly. "And she surrenders to me," he says. "She surrenders like she never has before, losing her senses, no longer thinking. She knows that I will bring her to a place she has never been to if only she agrees to lose control and follow me. She will realize that I am the best thing that ever happened to her . . . She'll let me touch her body. I can't stop thinking of her body." Danny speaks. I listen. "It's not me, it's him," he apologizes, and I know he talks about his fear of the ghost that possesses him and speaks from his throat, fear of not being able to remove this voice from his head. He asks me to help him get rid of what he calls "the *Dybbuk*."

In Jewish tradition, the *Dybbuk* (Possession) is a ghost, a spirit, that finds no place in heaven or in hell. It wanders around until it penetrates the body of a living sinner. The only prospect for the person's recovery is a traditional Chasidic ritual designed to convince the ghost to leave. But who is this ghost? And how much fear is involved in the encounter with ghosts and spirits that invade our lives and the therapeutic dyad?

In discussing Danny's case, I will touch upon our tendency as humans to think we must keep ghosts away, afraid of their unknown impact on our lives. The more traditional practices involve a haunting quest to expel ghosts and spirits, but at least ideally, psychoanalysis as well as the Chasidic tradition seek to invite them in first, wishing to get to know them.

Trying to become acquainted with the *Dybbuk* I met in the analytic treatment, I examine here the Chasidic tradition aimed at treating the *Dybbuk,* as well as traditional and modern modes of thought and treatment.

Ghosts hold for us parts of our history, shameful parts, scary parts, parts that need to be forgotten or that are denied access (Loewald, 1960). I will address the ghost that contains these parts of the self that are experienced as "not-me" and that take over the self. In Danny's case, the experience is of the *Dybbuk* as powerful and threatening, a force that might annihilate him and steal his "real" identity. I will discuss our *sins* as they are held by the sinner's ghost: Danny's sins, my sins, brutality, sexuality and psychoanalytic sins.

Dealing with the split between good and bad, right and wrong, reality and fantasy, I will revisit the "too muchness" (Atlas, 2014; Benjamin & Atlas, 2015), the experience of dysregulation, or as it has been called by Laplanche (1989; 1992; 1995), Stein (1998) and Benjamin (2004), Excess: more tension than is felt to be pleasurable or bearable. I will address the connection between sexuality and attachment, the seeking of regulation and containment and the solution of internal split between passive and active, when one part of the self is functioning as a container for the other part in order to resolve the problem of excess and failure of self-regulation.

The "bad" father and the tender witness

Danny grew up in Israel. He has five older sisters, so he is the youngest brother and only son. His parents divorced when he was seven, and he moved to live at his maternal grandparents' together with his mother and sisters. The relationship with his father was severely curtailed, and during the first years of therapy we worked through the separation from father, with whom Danny was so closely connected but also disappointed and angry. As a child, Danny and his father would spend hours together, building airplanes and playing in the yard. While Danny loved his father dearly, he was aware that the father was abusive toward his mother and feared his father's fits of anger. When his parents divorced, the children and their mother moved to a far-off town and rarely saw their father again.

In the first sessions Danny tells me that his father is a bad and cruel man, a monster, and that he himself is just like him. Soon enough we touch upon the pain of loss, the longing, and the significant object that Danny had lost. Danny says that the "good father" and the "bad father" could not coexist, and that the "bad father" won. Talking about the good father, we get in touch with the child that Danny had been: the loving, creative, mischievous child, the child who misses his father, the one who cries into his pillow at night without understanding why. This child is different from the way Danny presents himself as an adult. He is a man in his early thirties, an economist who lives alone and comes for treatment because he cannot create a meaningful relationship with a woman. He tells me that he is a rigid, strict man, and that he fears he is manipulative, exactly like his father. He says that he treats people like tools that he has to learn to handle. He warns me that he is critical, that he will probably think that I am stating the obvious, and that he will think that I am a bad dresser, "Because I have yet to meet a woman who knows how to dress," he says. When he says this I think about his interest in women's clothing. He is aware of what I am wearing in every session and therefore of what I am not wearing, which I take to be an attempt on Danny's part to cover women's naked bodies through a continual preoccupation with the unflattering clothes they wear. As for his sex life, he tells me dryly that there is no such thing.

I see Danny three times a week during the first year of therapy. Both of us are usually very serious. On rare occasions we laugh, a short, focused, almost cynical laugh. We talk about his father, his identification with the exploitative father, his fear that he is exactly like him—cruel and cold. The bad father who is imprinted in his memory, violent, abandoning, is the bad Danny as he currently experiences himself. Danny cries, recalls the good and beloved child, the good and beloved father, whom he had erased from memory so as not to experience the pain of separation and to lend meaning to the abandonment. He barely mentions his mother. She does not exist. She is an absent, dead mother (Green, 1983). I wonder if Danny is protecting her, as well as me, from his longing and anger. He says that he is afraid of his crazy parts, of irrationality.

We get to know the boy that Danny once was. "It is so strange to think that maybe there really is a little boy alive inside of me. He barely has any air," he says. And I agree, the child that resides within him is barred from entering the world, the adults' world. In one of the dreams that he presents there is a little boy, and he leads the boy by the hand to a small, dark room and tells him, "Wait here, don't move, don't go out, you'll be safe here." We talk about the child who is locked up in the room and understand that he wishes to protect the child from the pain, the violence, from life as he experiences it.

Elsewhere I wrote about the confusion of tongues that arises in the chasm and dialectic between the language of tenderness and the language of aggression, as it appears in the therapeutic relationship, and the way in which patient and therapist collude to avoid aggression (Atlas, 2010). This occurs to protect the tender parts that evolve in the co-constructed third of the treatment, and to prevent the retraumatization of both parties. Danny witnessed his father's brutality. He was afraid of his father and afraid he could be as brutal as him. Part of the process, especially when dealing with trauma, terror and helplessness, consists of an unconscious collusion or mutual "agreement" between therapist and patient—each of whom contains both a victim and an aggressor simultaneously (Davies & Frawley, 1992)—that the aggression poses a threat to each other and to the therapy. The collusion embodies an attempt to protect the tender and benevolent parts of the treatment, as well as the witness, in this case the witness that Danny once was, and me as a witness. Underneath there is always the fear that the witness will be destroyed by the trauma, or, as Sam Gerson writes, there is always fear of contamination (Gerson, 2009). Thus, we first need to make sure that we can protect our witness, whether it is the little boy that Danny needs to hide in the room or the witnessing parts that exist in the treatment, even though this protection is associated with the dissociation and denial that is co-experienced in the treatment. We collude to protect the one part from the anxiety-provoking other, defending against the terror of being traumatized through attack, penetration, humiliation and destruction.

Benjamin describes the core of male anxiety, whereby the penis is seen as hurtful to or destructive of the mother's body (Benjamin, 2009, personal communication). Danny is constantly afraid of his own masculinity. He cannot allow himself to be a man, but also has no access to the boy he once was. He is in limbo, just like a ghost who cannot find its place anywhere, and he feels that he must always be cautious. As a child Danny felt he needed to protect his mother not only from his "bad" father but also from her potentially bad son and from his intense feelings, especially his need and rage, that later on translated to sexual needs. The fear, then, is both of being destructive and of being destroyed. Danny tries to protect the scared little boy he is from the scary adult he is and I might be, but also from us as witnesses to what one can see but cannot bear. So we began therapy with a collusion, an unconscious agreement to protect that boy and the tender parts of the treatment and not let aggression or sexuality into the room. Only after a safe enough environment was created could the *Dybbuk* appear. "The Dybbuk came and ruined it all," Danny says.

Your heart must not be soft

The term *Dybbuk* originates from the Hebrew root *Dabak* (to attach, to cling). Observant Chasidim and Torah scholars are said to be *Dvekim BaTora,* which means that they attached or cling to the Torah and do not let go. Similarly, the *Dybbuk* is a ghost that takes over the person, clings without letting go, like *Devek*—glue. The *Dybbuk,* the soul of a sinful person who has been barred entry into heaven as well as hell, and which is also named an "evil spirit" in Talmudic literature, seeks its repair (*Tikun*). The Cabalists use the ritual in an attempt to get the ghost to talk and to engage it in conversation so as to understand who it is and why it has invaded the person's body. The goal is to remove the ghost from the person's body, thereby curing him from the *Dybbuk*. But this is no easy feat, the rabbis warn, since the ghost that wishes to remain within the person's body tends to cunningly conceal its identity. Tradition has it that the ghost speaks out from the person's mouth in a voice different from his, virtually without moving his lips, and tries to be misleading when one tries to reveal its identity. It often presents another person's identity so it can remain unidentified and forego expulsion. The goal is therefore to first identify the ghost and engage it in dialogue. It is claimed that the ghost then leaves through the little toe of the left foot and that in this state even amputating the toe will not cause the person any significant physical harm (Arica, 2001).

Rabbi Chaim Vital, a disciple of the mystic Rabbi Isaac Luria (*HaAri*), describes in his book *The Holy Ghost* how *HaAri* taught him to expel evil spirits: "I would take that man's arm and set my hand on his pulse . . . and while holding the pulse in my hand I would say the verse . . . and then he says anything you ask from within the body, and you order him to leave. And sometimes you must sound the *Shofar* (ram's horn) near his ear . . . " The rabbi instructs the ghost expeller to exorcise it using a certain incantation and by uttering Cabalists' names. He adds that one should "aim for all of the names to forcefully come out, and if they do not, repeat the mentioned verse and aim for all the mentioned names. And in the end always say forcefully, '*Tze', tze be- mehera!* [leave, leave quickly!]' And know that essentially, you must make your heart brave and strong like a hero, *with no fear,* and your heart must not be soft." In order to verify that the same ghost does not move into another Jewish body it must be excommunicated, "so that it will not cause harm and will not enter any Israelite whatsoever (Arica, 2001, my translation)."

Fear is the motif that is revisited time and again when dealing with ghosts. The rabbis warn that in cases where the ghost expeller is afraid, his mission is destined to fail. The goal is to succeed in meeting the ghost fearlessly. Danny keeps on warning me, "Don't get near there. If you meet the ghost, something terrible will happen." What happens then when we meet the *Dybbuk* in the analytic space? Can we let it in without feeling too threatened for our lives and by our own sins? Can we bear living with that which cannot be represented in words?

"For a few years the voice I heard was soft, so that I managed to fight it and silence it," Danny says. "But as time passed, its volume rose and rose until it became a loud voice that resounded not only in my head; I imagine everyone can hear it, and it takes over my actions, too. It might make me do horrible things if I stop fighting it." Danny refers to the terrible things he might do to women, and especially his obsession over Leah, his dream girl, who didn't pay attention to him because "she knows to choose between good and bad."

After a year of therapy, the *Dybbuk* entered the room and its voice became louder to my ears, too. It expressed desire mixed with hostility and frustration, along with the scary feeling that all these are out of Danny's control. Danny was afraid of his acts. For moments I feared it too, especially when Danny told me directly that he might harm me. He repeatedly said that he has no control over the *Dybbuk* and that therefore he cannot tell what he might do. But many other times I couldn't tell if I was afraid or excited, and which of these was a defense against the other. From an early age I learned to overcome fears, especially because I was afraid most of the time. My father taught me to charge forward when I'm afraid, just like in combat, to try to go on marching while making sure I keep thinking. With Danny, in moments when I feel the fear, I ask myself what we are actually afraid of. Is it lack of control? The unknown? Aggression? Sexuality? His sins? My sins? Insanity? There were moments when I scolded myself for not being afraid enough, for being too curious, wanting more. I asked myself whether I was actively experiencing everything that Danny could not allow himself to feel—the excitement, the curiosity, the passion—leaving him passive, overstimulated and anxious. This is when I first start feeling like a sinner.

It's me or him

"Why do you take me so seriously?" Danny was skeptical at times. "Do you actually believe in ghosts and spirits?!" he asked. "Maybe I'm simply schizophrenic . . . Say, deep inside, don't you think all of this is bizarre? Suddenly we're here talking about this *Dybbuk* as if it was really rational, something that exists. And yet it is so real, so powerful. So scary." I recall myself as a young girl telling my two best friends that we must hold a séance to conjure the spirits of the dead, convincing them until they agree, because surely a good spirit would come and save me, teach me something I did not know.

A few decades later, I realize the same fantasy is propelling me: To get to know the ghost that will teach me something spectacular and that will be a savior from a life of death, of devastation. I understand that I experience Danny the way I used to experience my mother: As not fully alive, in limbo between child and adult, between being alive and being dead. And when I am with him, I feel like the girl I was, who is afraid that if she shuts her eyes and then reopens them, she will discover that she was right, and that she really is completely alone in the world—just like he discovered when he separated from his father.

Danny says, "This is crazy. It's totally illogical. I can't understand why you go on talking like that, as though I were talking logically, as though I wasn't nuts. As if you believe every word I say. Only unrealistic people really believe that there is such a thing, a *Dybbuk*. I drive it out of my head, and it comes back. You and I talk irrationally," Danny summarizes decisively, pointing at the split between us: I'm active, he is passive, I "go on talking like that . . . " while he is being penetrated by the *Dybbuk*. At those moments I fear that I might be violating some basic psychoanalytic rule. Here again, I'm the sinner, I think. Maybe he is right and I am letting something dangerous and forbidden happen. I'm allowing the ghost to come in. I'm allowing the forbidden thought and feelings to enter the room. We are dealing with "rules"—psychoanalytic rules, Jewish rules, ethical rules, rules that split between good and bad, right and wrong, dangerous and safe, and of course between a sinner and a saint, shame and pride.

A battle between what Danny calls the "good ones and the bad ones" is taking place. "And it's clear who's going to win," he says, "You know Leonard Cohen's song? It goes like this: *"Everybody knows that the dice are loaded, Everybody rolls with their fingers crossed, Everybody knows the war is over, Everybody knows the good guys lost."* "It's so accurate," Danny says. "Only kids believe that the good guys always win."

And so we have good ones and bad ones. There is "me" and "not-me." And we continually talk about sins. There is a part that sins and a part that must remain pure, with no dialogue between them. One is a threat to the other.

In psychoanalysis, the term "not-me" was first used by Sullivan (1953) when he outlined good-me, bad-me, and not-me states.[1] Bromberg considers "not me" to be a normal function of the human mind, which is ubiquitous in every human relationship and asks, "Why should one part of oneself be terrified of meeting another part? How does a *person* come to feel 'haunted?'" (Bromberg, 2003, p. 687). He writes that the "not me" is a ghost that not only evokes fear, it also generates *shame* when it emerges in the patient-therapist relationship (Chefetz & Bromberg, 2004). With reference to dissociative experiences, Bromberg views dreams as partly manifesting not-me experiences. In analyzing a dream, we have the opportunity to help the patient listen to otherwise dissociated self states and begin to link between them (2006). Altman (1995) writes that the "other" often becomes a receptacle for not-me projections and is then shunned or feared.

The ghost, then, can be understood as the shameful not-me part of the self, which cannot be represented in words and projected onto the scary other. Bromberg writes: "The analyst's making optimal use of dissociative processes in an intersubjective and interpersonal context enables the patient more readily to self-regulate affect in those areas of implicit memory where trauma has left its mark; the dissociated ghosts of 'not-me' are thus persuaded, little by little, to cease their haunting and participate more and more actively and openly as self-reflective, self-expressive parts of 'me'" (Bromberg, 2003, p. 689).

In Chasidism, the method of "evoking the alien thoughts" (Arzy, Fachler, & Kahana, 2004) is meant to create a dialogue between the rational world and what people define as the irrational; between the known world and the clandestine one, the permissible and the prohibited, life and death, and what we understand to be different self states. The goal then is not to get rid of "alien thoughts" that "do not belong to me," but rather to identify their roots. Not to expel the *Dybbuk,* but to ask it to come out so that we can get to know its face. In order to do so we must ask, "Who are you?"

Without your clothes

"Here, I'm about to come. I come and hope that I've gotten rid of it, that now I'm free, since my semen is outside and this *Dybbuk* that's persecuting me persistently has been expelled. I look at it—a stain on a towel. There, I've finished it off. It's not inside me anymore. I've won. That's what I think. But then I hear a whisper . . . and she reappears. Leah—pretty, clothed, pure." Danny and I begin talking about the clothes. "What is she wearing?" I ask. Danny describes her white dress, the narrow straps, the delicate material. "You describe her clothed, while I imagine her nude," I say. "Interesting," he answers. "I'll tell you something that happened when I was nine or ten. My sisters would walk around the house naked. They were already adolescents, and boys would come home and they would go to their rooms with them and shut the door. One day I walked past my sister's room and she sat there in a long-sleeved shirt, legs spread apart. 'Why are you wearing black underwear?' I asked her, and she burst out laughing wildly. Clearly she was not wearing any underwear. It became the family joke. *I* became the family joke. And although deep inside I knew she was naked, I'm not sure why it was important for me to hide it and pretend she was wearing underwear." "Maybe you hoped she was wearing underwear?" I asked. "I still hope so," he laughs, and I say, "You hope all women are dressed, that you won't face them in the nude and re-experience your childhood experience."

The ghosts and the spirits; the dark world in Jewish mythology (Dagan, 2003), is linked with sins and sexuality. The spirits, for example, are considered to be created through masturbation. After the first sin and expulsion from the Garden of Eden, the spirits slept with Adam and with Eve for 130 years, and ghosts, spirits, and Liliths—part human, part ghost— were born. The ghosts were associated with blood, that is, aggression, but especially with sex and anything related to sexual activity, including what were considered to be lustful thoughts. The first female ghost, Lilith, is considered to have been created with Adam, before Eve. Adam could not stand her power, and particularly her sexual power when she insisted on being on top when they had sex. He therefore asked God to get rid of her and to create another, docile woman. Another female ghost named Askara was an expert in extorting lustful thoughts from people. The ghosts and the spirits grew and gained in power from semen ejaculated for mere pleasure—that is, not for impregnation. It was claimed that above all they loved detached sex that is not part of an intimate relationship (Dagan, 2003).

The ghosts are bound with a dead man who had sinned and they invade the body of a live person that has an opening; not necessarily a person who has already sinned but someone who is prone to sin. The Cabalists' role is to try and extract the ghost from the person's body and to identify who it is and why it entered him. When the person turns his head to the wall, the ghost can speak from inside him and describe why it was punished. The punishment is usually associated with sex, a punishment for adultery or other lecherous acts. When the live person acknowledges the impiety and regrets it, the rabbi sentences the ghost to expulsion and orders it to leave through the little toe of the left foot.

Hartman's study on the *Dybbuk* (1987) is based on an analysis of 63 cases over 400 years. The author discusses spirit possession in terms of individual motivation and societal restraints. He found that the *Dybbuk* idiom provided a means by which forbidden sexual wishes could be symbolized and expressed in a way that decreased their threat both for the individual and for the community.

Excess and containment, longing and shame

Danny and I understand that he is dealing with the shameful child that he was and still is. We start addressing the connection between sexuality and attachment, and touch Danny's shameful longing for the maternal body, the clothes as representing remnants of the maternal skin that he is not allowed to want. The need then, creates much shame. Danny's experience is of being overwhelmed and abandoned; his mother is absent. Women shame him and might expose his physical and emotional needs and longings. The sisters represent the exciting feminine body, and this generates the experience of excess—more tension than is felt to be pleasurable or even bearable, particularly by the immature psyche (Benjamin, 2004; Laplanche, 1989, 1992, 1995; Stein, 1998). Danny seeks regulation, must shut his eyes so as not to do something forbidden, to refrain from thinking and feeling something prohibited: his own sexual arousal, longing and shame.

Danny tries to regulate the tension through bodily discharge, when he masturbates and hopes that he has now "gotten rid of it." But he cannot get rid of this part of himself. Benjamin writes that discharge when detached from the aim of enjoying the other or coming in contact with another mind, indicates the use of the body to solve the problem mental excess (Benjamin, 2004). Danny experiences the excitement and stimulation as "too much" and is afraid of being active ("I'll become my father, I'll do something terrible, forbidden, dangerous").

We are dealing here then with the problem of tension and excess within an intersubjective framework. There is a failure of self-regulation based on deficient responses by the other—responses variously conceptualized as holding, containment and mentalization. This failure, initially an intersubjective one, generates the experience of excess. Danny's experience is of being overwhelmed and abandoned. According to Benjamin (2004), the problem of excess can generate a split between activity and passivity. The boy's experience leads him to seek an object that can contain the excitement and take the place of passivity. Benjamin writes that the boy establishes his own activity by projecting the experience of being passive onto the girl, creating the split between active and passive, masculine and feminine. As I will discuss, in Danny's case the split between passive and active is internal. One part of the self is functioning as a container for the other part in order to resolve the problem of excess and failure of self-regulation.

Danny's childhood solution is to remain passive and have the *Dybbuk* be the sinner. The *Dybbuk* holds the dissociative, threatening part, the not-me. He is active while Danny is penetrated by him. I believe that since he had not experienced the passive function of mother as container, an internal split is happening. He becomes the container for his own mind. Corrigan & Gordon (1995) following Winnicott's concept of the "Premature ego development" (1949, 1951) defined the "mind object", when the mind is cathected as an object that omnipotently attempts to replace the caretaking environment, it's the tendency in early development to turn prematurely away from the mother and toward the mind instead. The mind then replaces the object as an adaptation to the intersubjective failure and as an attempt to solve the problem of "wanting" and the shameful needs of the mind and body. In Danny's case we see how through the split of the mind, one part of the self is functioning as a container for the other, "not-me" part. One is passive, the other is active. Danny is the passive innocent; the *Dybbuk* the active sinner.

Conclusion

We began therapy with a collusion, the unconscious agreement to protect the tender parts of ourselves and the treatment and not let aggression or sexuality into the room. Only after a safe enough environment was created could the *Dybbuk* appear, and I hear Danny's fantasy about Leah as his communication with me as well: His sexual fantasy, the fear his sexual and emotional need will leak and he won't be able to control himself, the fantasy that I will submit to him, allow something forbidden to happen. In many ways, I'm his oldest sister who is sitting in front of him with no underwear and he has to pretend he doesn't see, can't let himself notice that I'm a woman, and can't allow himself to feel he needs me. My sexuality creates disregulation and repeats his childhood experience, which can only be dissociated. Later on, when we develop the symbolic language that represents his childhood experience, we are able to maintain the "as if" and talk about the sexuality in the room without reliving his childhood overexcitement and disregulation. The *Dybbuk*'s voice weakens. Danny gradually treats it as expressing parts of himself. One day he comes in smiling and tells me that he has asked Leah to go out with him. She agreed.

Note

1 The good-me is everything we like about ourselves. It represents the part of us we share with others and that we often choose to focus on because it produces no anxiety. The bad-me represents those aspects of the self that are considered negative and are therefore hidden from others, and possibly even from the self. The not-me represents all those things that are so anxiety-provoking that we cannot even consider them a part of us. It is kept out of awareness by pushing it deep into the unconscious.

An earlier version of this chapter was originally published in the book *The Enigma of Desire: Sex, Longing and Belonging in Psychoanalysis*, by Galit Atlas, Routledge, 2015, and is reprinted by permission of Taylor & Francis, LLC.

Bibliography

Altman, N. (1995). *The Analyst in the Inner City: Race, Class, and Culture Through a Psychoanalytic Lens.* New York, NY: Relational Perspectives Book Series.
Arica, Y. (2001). *Reincarnation: Reality that Exceeds All Imagination.* Kfar Sava: Aryeh Nir Publications, Ltd.
Arzy, S., Fachler, B. & Kahana, B. (2004). *Life as a Midrash. Perspectives in Jewish Psychology.* Tel Aviv: Yediot.
Atlas, G. (2010). Confusion of Tongues: Trauma and Playfulness. *Psychoanalytic Perspectives*, 6 (2): 93–114.
Atlas, G. (2015). Touch me, Know me: The Enigma of Desire. In, *The Enigma of Desire: Sex, Longing and Belonging in Psychoanalysis.* New York, NY: Routledge.
Benjamin, J. (2004). Revisiting the Riddle of Sex. In I. Matthis (Ed.), *Dialogues on Sexuality, Gender and Psychoanalysis* (pp. 145–172). London: Karnac.
Benjamin, J. (2009). Personal communication.
Benjamin, J. & Atlas, G. (2015). The "Too Muchness" of Excitement: Sexuality in Light of Excess, Attachment and Affect Regulation. *The International Journal for Psychoanalysis.* Feb, 96 (1) 39–63.

Bromberg, P.M. (2003). One Need Not Be a House to Be Haunted. *Psychoanal. Dial.*, 13: 689–709.

Bromberg, P. (2006). *Awakening the Dreamer: Clinical Journeys*. Hillsdale, NJ: The Analytic Press.

Chefetz, R.A., & Bromberg, P.M. (2004). Talking with "Me" and "Not-Me." *Contemp. Psychoanal.*, 40: 409–464.

Corrigan, E. & Gordon, P. (1995). *The Mind Object: Precocity and Pathology of Self-Sufficiency*. Northvale, NJ: Jason Aronson.

Dagan, H. (2003). *Jewish Mythology*. Tel Aviv: Map.

Davies, J.M., & Frawley, M.G. (1992). Dissociative Processes and Transference Countertransference Paradigms in the Psychoanalytically Oriented Treatment of Adult Survivors of Childhood Sexual Abuse. *Psychoanal. Dial.*, 2: 5–36.

Freud. S. (1932). Female Sexuality. *Int. J. Psycho-Anal.*, 13: 281–297.

Gerson, S. (2009). When the Third Is dead: Memory, Mourning, and Witnessing in the Aftermath of the Holocaust. *Int. J. Psychoanal.* 90: 1341–1357.

Green, A. (1983). The Dead Mother. In *On Private Madness*. London: Hogarth Press, pp. 142–73.

Hartman, J.J. (1987). Psychoanalytic Study of Society, XI,. *Psychoanal Q.*, 56: 737.

Laplanche, J. (1989). *New Foundations for Psychoanalysis*. (Trans. D. Macey). Oxford, UK: Basil Blackwell.

―――― (1992). *Seduction, Translation, Drives*. Ed. J. Fletcher & M. Stanton. Institute of Contemporary Arts, London.

―――― (1995). Seduction, Persecution and Revelation. *Int. J. Psychoanal.*, 76: 663–682.

Loewald, H.W. (1960). On the Therapeutic Action of Psycho-Analysis. *Int. J. Psycho-Anal.*, 41: 16–33

Stein, R. (1998). The Poignant, the Excessive and the Enigmatic in Sexuality. *Int. J. Psychoanal.*, 79: 253–268.

Stoller, R.J. (1974). Hostility and Mystery in Perversion. *Int. J. Psycho-Anal.*, 55: 425–434.

Sullivan, H. S. (1953). *The Interpersonal Theory of Psychiatry*. New York, NY: Norton.

Winnicott, D.W. (1949). Mind and its Relation to the Psyche-soma. In: *Collected Papers*. London: Hogarth, 1958, pp. 243–254.

Winnicott, D. W. (1951). Transitional Objects and Transitional Phenomena. In: *Through Paediatrics to Psycho-Analysis: Collected Papers*. New York, NY: Brunner/Mazel, 1992, pp. 229–242.

Chapter 3

Occupation
A ghost story

Arthur Fox

"I was in the barber shop with my friends. I was about 14. My friends were looking at the *Playboys*. I couldn't. I knew that if I looked, my mom would find out. She would see it in my mind the minute I walked in the door. There was no way I could get that past her."

This is 10 minutes into Richard's first consultation with me. He stares at me hollow-eyed. He can see that I am mesmerized: The predicament he's remembering from his adolescence—a beloved and angry parent will catch him with a sexual thought, and he has no protection from the burning shameful exposure, no privacy—it sounds odd to me. But also familiar in a way that I am not eager to think about.

Richard has come for a consultation saying "I am not depressed I don't think, but I don't feel like I am really in my life. At some point I sort of lost myself—I think I got cut off from my 'Eros'" (he makes air quotes with his fingers). In this first hour, I am feeling a little lost also. There is a funny mix of friendliness and forboding in Richard: he addresses me as "Art"; he tells me my card was on his desk for two years before he got around to calling. And my unease about Richard's Eros is drawing up a worry about my own: Richard seems to match a type I have always been drawn to—highly disciplined Irish Catholic guys who seem to be able to talk about their misery without being crippled by it—guys who seem to err on the side of needing too little. And now meeting with Richard for the first time, I am finding myself embarrassingly excited as he tells me about his family life: "I have a great life: great wife and three wonderful kids— I know I love them dearly, and that I need them, but I can't really seem to FEEL any of it."

I am thinking about choked-back love, and he seems to read it in my face. He keeps talking: "whatever it is that is making me so cut off—I think it also has to do with the fact that I was anorexic when I was about 12. It lasted a year and a half. I had no idea what made me stop eating. I just had to. I asked my mom to take me to a therapist and she did. And I just sat there saying nothing. I went for three sessions just saying nothing. I remember thinking that he was listening, really trying to get inside me. But something made me sit there and not talk." His face lightens up "I sort of feel bad for the guy."

He goes on: "I think it has to do with my mother. Growing up, I always had the sense that she knew something about me that was too human. Not good. I joke sometimes that I don't have a conscience; I have my mother in my mind, watching what I am doing and feeling and thinking. Everything that happens in my mind is put before her for review, and her judgment is absolute, infallible, ex cathedra." More embarrassed excitement as I notice that he's trusting me to know what that means.

I ask about this phrase "too human." Richard looks at me intently, as if he's wondering about this word for the first time. Then he says "For some reason I am thinking about my grandmother, my mother's mother who I never knew. She had to go back to Ireland to take care of some sick relative, and never came home. I think my mom was around 11 when she left." He goes on, the determination in his face fading to a kind of blankness: "It wasn't like my mother never talked about her mother when we were growing up," Richard says. "But when she did, there was always this quality of evanescence. You never had the sense that my mom missed her now, or had even missed her or been angry or mourned her in some way when she left."

This is seeming like a lot of information for a first consultation. And there's more. At the time of his onset of anorexia, an older brother had dropped out of college. "My parents said he had depression but I thought he had anorexia also and was hiding it. He had moved back in with us and sort of never left his bedroom. I remember hearing my mom upstairs crying trying to get him to come down and have dinner." I ask for other memories of the time of onset. "It was spring. Swimming pre-season was underway; the coach was talking to me about being scouted for scholarships, I was a national merit scholar . . . " Friends? I ask. "Yeah actually. I had a serious girlfriend. I think I loved her but I felt like I had no idea whatsoever what I wanted from her. We'd be downstairs in the rec room making out, and I remember her making it clear that she wanted more, but I had no idea what I wanted."

At this point in the consultation I notice that I am fighting off an awareness that Richard's story—ostensibly about missing Eros—is actually being presented to me as a story about conflicted sexuality: Anorexia and sexual numbness in a sensitive straight male adolescent (and the long pre-relationship with my business card)? My eyes fall heavily on his forearms—they are gym-built, tattooed. Suddenly I notice that the song from Popeye the Sailor has started looping in my mind. I struggle to make it stop but it keeps on repeating, mocking him, mocking me mocking him. I feel my face flushing; it feels like a listening mask. I am too scared and embarrassed to wonder if I am actually living, in this moment, a close mimic of the feeling of helpless shaming exposure that made Richard know he had to avoid the *Playboys*.

This is Richard's third try at therapy. Neither previous effort lasted more than six months. "I didn't feel like I was getting anywhere," he says. But he takes easily to the work with me, and the first weeks of the treatment are full of memories and stories and "a sense that something is breaking loose in me, something is being freed up." I am feeling increasingly the opposite: I find myself locked in a markedly unanalytic state of mind when I am with him. Nearly everything Richard says or does gets slapped into the same schema: This is a case of internalized homophobia. Richard feels distanced from his life because some early and fundamental object choice—probably a homosexual one—is being censored by his mother as she lives inside his mind. There's a ghost where Richard's superego should be, a mother who is "holding" what Richard refers to as his Eros, who threatens to excoriate him with shame if he feels excitement about his body or another person's. The Popeye the Sailor song keeps cropping up obnoxiously in my reverie. Why? Is this my unconscious telling me to listen to Richard's semiotics rather than his words? Is it a wish to counter-humiliate Richard's homophobic censors? Maybe simply a wish to engage him in a way that feels less brittle? Maybe just spoiling, mocking envy? My self-inquiry gets me nowhere and in the first few months I feel, in the sessions with Richard, like I am being held by a choke-collar both to the idea of Richard's internalized homophobia, and to my own shame about being unable to get that idea out of my mind.

Six months into the treatment Richard starts feeling depressed. "A feeling of loss that I can't put my finger on." Watching his son play soccer he feels a sudden unbearable sadness remembering himself at 12. Richard realizes that this depression is getting him somewhere and he increases to twice a week. I see the tension fall from his face as he begins each session. I feel gratified that something is happening to Richard that hasn't happened before. But my ability to listen with equanimity, to keep an analytic attitude, isn't getting any better. I have a creepy sense that I am up to no good, that I am overfocused on ferreting out a sexual ambivalence buried deep inside Richard. Even my preoccupation with my own glitches in analytic functioning feels corrupt.

Richard begins to worry about his dependence on me and the treatment. "I feel that I am coming undone," he says. His internist prescribes an antidepressant, and Richard begins to report an intensity of love for his wife and sons that's new. He notices that he is fascinated by his younger son's unselfconsciousness physical grace and confidence. Even his older son's peevishness and pot smoking make him feel like there is something opening up inside him—"I am sort of remembering what it was like for me. I can see myself at his age and feel something like I am ok and HE is ok too."

Richard tapers off his antidepressant and the depression resurges. He says he feels more at home in his life, but there is still a sense of overwhelming sadness about the love he feels for his family—"I can see it right there in front of me, but its so fragile. Evanescent. I feel it and then it's gone. Like waking from a dream and forgetting it." Fourteen months in, Richard announces that work is slow—he is a filmmaker, and the commercial projects that pay the bills have dried up. He has to terminate treatment. I feel a rush of shame (I have been charging him my full fee, twice a week. How could I have overlooked the signs that he is running out of money?) Impulsively I say: "No, we're not done. I say we continue to meet twice a week at a fee of 40 dollars until work picks up for you." He agrees but there's a change. The next week he says: "I have come as far as I want to. This will be my last session. And don't take this the wrong way but I hope you can fill my hours with someone who can actually pay your fee." I know I should be insulted by this but I can't quite figure out why. I recover enough to say: "It sounds like you're worried about a dependence I might have on YOU. I think you've taken on the role of your mother, who lived by the rule: Don't ever become emotionally dependent on someone; people leave."

It's a Hail-Mary interpretation and I know it won't take. And even though I think it's right, it feels wrong—desperate, glib—and I am left feeling like I am the one asking for too much from someone who is fine without me.

But Richard agrees to come back next week. Over the weekend he attends a cousin's wedding and on the Monday he comes in a changed man: "At the wedding I looked over at Inga and the boys and realized that there was a real goodness there, that I don't have to worry so much about what I do or don't think I feel—that I don't have to think about everything so much. So thank you for all your help and this will be our last session." He stares at me, still gaunt, still hollow-eyed. We look at each other quietly for three or four minutes. "I would probably continue this," he says, "if I didn't feel like I was being attacked for being a psychotherapy patient every time I leave your office." The silence, then this, have left me a little bit stunned. It's the end of the hour and I have no comeback. In fact, at the moment, quitting feels to me like its the right thing for Richard to do: I find myself agreeing, internally, that whatever it is that Richard stands to gain from continuing treatment is going to be less good—emotionally, morally—than what he already has and stands to lose. Which is what? A sense of being decent? An ability to not live in fear of internal surprise attack?

So why is this a ghost story?

I like the word Ghost because it creates a link between something that we talk about in psychoanalysis—unmetabolized objects, created in intergenerational transmission of trauma and unmourned losses, sustained by dissociation—and something that, every kid in the world knows—feels in his bones—is real, and scary. Ghosts are menacing and powerful. They show up suddenly and then vanish before one has evidence of their existence, leaving one alone, scared and doubting one's own experience. A good ghost story draws its listeners in, undoes them and holds them bound anxiously hoping for resolution and release. And ghosts can haunt in many ways—a panic attack, a shame attack or a sudden onslaught of guilt or despair. To a child, a ghost is like a bad parent: Magically powerful, but also erratic. They are a part of you; they live inside your world but you can never learn enough about them to make them less scary. This is why I like the word Ghost—because in life there are things that it is appropriate to be afraid of. And when we use a term like unmetabolized bad object, we might get a feeling that we know what we're talking about.

In trying to understand what went wrong in the treatment with Richard I went back to the books to think about what exactly is an unmetabolized object. The most compelling explanation I found was from Freudians like

Loewald (1973), who basically say that they're failed internalizations. Failed in the sense that a real-life pre-oedipal parent gets demolished and broken up into it's constituent affective parts—the scary, the soothing, the wonderously good and the scathingly critical—but rather than being absorbed—metabolized—into the ego and becoming structures, they remain something like free radicals in the personality. Terror, idealization, shame—aspects of what parents look like to young children, preserved in all their original fairy-taleish supernatural power.

I think this is what Richard was describing when he said that his mother was in his head, exercising an all-powerful censorship of some part of his humanity that had to do with pleasure in love. What he wanted me to understand was that it didn't feel like a superego—a part of *him* that generated feelings of right and wrong and thus motivated him this way or that way. Instead it felt like a kind of occupation—a homeland lockdown by a foreign power that is all-powerful and invisible.

Bion (1962) tells us that emotional experiences that haven't been metabolized—haven't undergone alpha function and become workable as dream thoughts or memories—can only be dealt with by projection. And I think projective identification is probably the most straightforward way of thinking about the weird complicity that came over me during Richard's last moments in my office: The ghost that had been seizing up Richard's Eros was now excoriating mine. This seems right but it doesn't explain why, from very early in Richard's treatment, I was so relentlessly focused on this as a story of conflict around sexuality rather than one of intergenerational transmission of trauma.

That question—why was I so fixed on the internalized homophobia hypothesis rather than the starvation and deadness—is particularly vexing to me because the idea of Richard that lingers in my mind now, three years after he quit, is not the one in my office with the muscles and tattoos. What I remember is the agony in his voice the night he called me crying—he'd had a moment of "total total despair" watching his youngest son at a swim meet. Over the phone, at night, Richard talked about a feeling of emptiness, and a dreadful sense that his son, now nearly adolescent, is soon going to notice inside himself the same ancient wordless devastation that Richard feels. Richard found that his hours with me—and occasionally my voice over the phone—provided some comfort from the pain and confusion of his depression. I think he came to love me for providing this for him. And I think it was that more pre-oedipal, dependant love—rather than a frankly erotic one—which made him the target of his mother's ghost's attacks—"she knew something about me that was too human, not good."

But why was it that at the last moment of the treatment, when Richard said exactly this to me—that what made therapy impossible was "feeling attacked" every time he left my office—why couldn't I speak? Roy Schafer (2003) has used the term "colonization" to describe states where the patient "invades and takes possession of the analyst's remembering." Remembering why Richard had come to therapy was exactly what I was unable to do during that final few minutes: Something was making me too scared to think as Richard's therapist. Instead, all I could feel was a sense that Richard and his morally tyrannical mother were right, and that I had been wrong to try to come between them. But maybe the idea of remembering and not remembering who you are in your work and in your history goes deeper than that.

Winnicott tells us that when we're dealing with our patient's depression what we're actually always dealing with is our patient's *mother's* depression (1971). This is something like what Henri Rey (1998) seems to be saying in his paper about what patients bring to analysis—a wish to repair their internal objects. Adrienne Harris (2009) has extended this idea of internal repair to what motivates analysts to do the work we do. The wish to heal some blighted but beloved early figure who lives inside of us, and the omnipotence to believe we can heroically swoop in and do that repair, is part of what sustains us through the difficulties of this work. But, Harris points out, repairing or relinquishing our ties to these objects can be extraordinarily difficult work, and our internal impasses often are implicated in impasses with our patients:

> The analyst's omnipotence, organized in the service of managing shame and envy, is a crucial block to grieving because in the omnipotent stance, there is no loss, no absence. Need itself seems to have been vanquished. In clinical instances of impasse, then, it is the potential for or barrier to grieving that lives alongside, in parallel and also distinct from these potentials in the patient. Since omnipotence blocks both grieving and the re-experience of shame and since there is pragmatic and real-life potential use of omnipotence in professional identities, the analyst's defensive stance in which omnipotence is prominent can be highly tenacious and resistant to movement.

What Harris is describing here is, I think, a situation where the therapist in the mere act of being a therapist elides aspects of his own experience that he needs access to in order to help his patient work through his own. This is a useful way of thinking about why Richard's mother's depression was sometimes outside the realm of full imaginability for me.

My grandparents on both sides escaped from Europe in the 1930s. My parents were adolescents in 1945, when the stories of the death camps started showing up in the morning papers and evening news broadcasts. This changed my parents. I think that without fully knowing it, they became people who had lost what Sam Gerson (2009) refers to as "a belief in a world that cares." I remember how their faces looked when they talked to me, as an adolescent in the 1970s, about what had happened to their families back in Europe. And I remember feeling, in a shameful and utterly secret way, like something inside them, and maybe inside me, had been ruined.

A Palestinian patient told me that he constantly struggles to keep from "falling into the pit of shame that comes from seeing yourself as a member of one of History's conquered peoples." Sam Gerson writes about what happens to historical memory when the historical facts of trauma are remembered, but the actual psychic damage is left unwitnessed:

> Even when trauma's initial impact of eluding representation is attenuated, the trauma, like a virulent virus, may evolve into a secrecy occasioned by the shame and guilt of being simultaneously within the gates of hell and living an everyday life.
>
> (2009)

There was depression in my family when I was growing up. But it was never linked in any way with history. There was constant talk of the Holocaust and Israel, but the shame of being a victim of history was not something you could talk or think about. Like Richard avoiding the pictures from the barber shop magazines, I had an inchoate sense that if I let a thought like that be alive in my mind, I'd be under intrapsychic attack the minute I walked in the front door.

Secret shame and the flight from secret shame may be where Richard's story intersects with mine. I think that my fascination with Catholics and Catholicness may have an element of flight from a deeper feeling of what it means to be a Jew in history. Catholicness, in my mind, has a sort of equivalence with unruinedness. Another type of unmetabolized preoedipal object—this one an idealization—one that apparently had to be exported outside Judaism to stay plausible. Like a lot of idealizations it doesn't hold up very well to reality testing. I would probably have been over it by age 15 if I hadn't kept it a secret.

Conclusion

History is a nightmare from which I am trying to awake.

I always assumed that it was a Jew who originally said that but it's actually from *Ulysses*. The Jews and the Irish seem to have something in common here. For me, what defines a nightmare is surprise: Something happens that you don't expect, can't protect yourself from and don't know how to stop. In the case of me and Richard, the nightmare traffic was shame attacks. Mine, I think, were related to big-H history and how it got encoded in my parents. Richard's I think had more to do with little-H—his mother's abandonment by her own mother, and a determination to survive it by killing off eros. (I imagine there was Big-H history in Richard's family as well; he never mentioned anything about famine, or immigration. And as philosophical as he was, he never shared a thought about adolescent anorexia as a meaningful symptom in an Irish American family.) Richard came to treatment (again, this was his third try as an adult) to try to get some understanding of something in him that was snuffing out his ability to feel love. I don't know what went wrong the first two times, but when he fled the treatment with me, I think it was because a renegade element of what should have been his superego had been stirred, and was ready to shame-stun either or both of us if we dared to feel dependence on, or loving gratitude toward, someone who was helping us grow. I was unable, at the time, to accept that in order to understand Richard's internal damage, I would need to have greater ability to think with my own mind about my own. Harris (2009) talks about this:

> Beyond the now conventional idea about countertransference as a kind of situational illness, we need to see the inevitable presence in the analyst of wounds that must serve as tools, aspects of the analyst's capacities that are simultaneously brakes on and potentials for change.

Papers on psychoanalytic process are not supposed to be scary. But ghost stories aren't good unless they *are* scary. In my experience as a psychotherapist, there are few things as scary as post-mortem examinations of premature terminations. When a patient forgoes their investment of time, pain and money because of, or partly because of, some defect in my work, it scares me: It forces me to think about what I don't know about the patient, about myself, and about what happened between us. As I started out writing about what happened to me in the work with Richard, I didn't know that it would turn out to be a story about how my clandestine shame—and shame *about* shame—colluded with Richard's in scuttling his treatment. But as that idea came to organize the story, I had a feeling that the occupying powers—mine, at least—were gradually being apprehended, and that the feelings that they were choking off were gradually being allowed out. When Loewald said "Those who know ghosts tell us that they long to be released from their ghost life and led to rest as ancestors," I think he was talking about something like this.

References

Bion, Wilfred (1962). *Learning from Experience*. London: Tavistock.
Gerson, S. (2009). When the Third is Dead: Memory Mourning and Witnessing in the Aftermath of the Holocaust. *International Journal of Psychoanalysis*, 90: 1341–1357.
Harris, Adrienne (2009). You Must Remember This. *Psychoanalytic Dialogues*, 19: 2–21.
Loewald, H.W. (1960). On the Therapeutic Action of Psycho-Analysis. *International Journal of Psychoanalysis*, 41: 16–33.
Loewald, H.W. (1973). On Internalization. *International Journal of Psychoanalysis*. 54: 9–17.
Rey, J.H. (1998). That Which Patients Bring to Analysis. *International Journal of Psychoanalysis*, 69: 457–470.
Schafer, Roy (2003) *Insight and Interpretation*. New York, NY: Other Press.
Winnicott, D.W. (1971). Mirror-role of Mother and Family in Child Development. In *Playing and Reality*, p. 155. New York, NY: Routledge.

Chapter 4

Repressed ghosts and dissociated vampires in the enacted dimension of psychoanalytic treatment

Gil Katz

Introduction

The universality of ghost stories and the enduring popularity of vampire movies and novels in contemporary culture is of course understandable psychoanalytically: ghosts and vampires (as well as the many other undead figures of myth and lore, such as zombies, shamblers, ghouls, revenants, dybbuks, and so on) are representations—projections and externalizations—of internally unacceptable impulses, early unresolved and conflictual object ties, and frightening psychic traumas.

The undead have also populated our psychoanalytic literature. Psychoanalytic Electronic Publishing's database currently lists 3,348 articles that contain references to ghosts and 471 that contain references to vampires. One of the most evocative uses of the metaphor of a ghost in psychoanalytic theory was crafted by Hans Loewald in his 1960 paper, "On the Therapeutic Action of Psycho-Analysis." In this seminal work, Loewald likened the process of psychoanalytic change to that of transforming psychic ghosts into ancestors.

In this chapter, I would like to supplement the metaphor of *ghosts that haunt* with the metaphor of *vampires that menace*. I will link these alien experiences to different psychological processes—repression and dissociation—and elaborate how both the ghosts and the vampires of a patient return to life within the *enacted dimension* of the treatment (Katz 1998, 2002, 2011, 2014). I will next discuss the process by which these unintegrated experiences may be assimilated into one's personality—transformed into ancestors—which I will illustrate with an extended clinical vignette in which the metaphor of a vampire figured prominently.

Two spectral metaphors

In psychoanalytic treatment, Loewald suggested, we engage the unintegrated internal objects who dwell in the unconscious and haunt present-day life—the ghosts of the past—in order to finally lay them to rest as ancestors. Once integrated into the fabric of the patient's psychic structure, these ancestors no longer haunt and distort contemporary relationships, but instead provide energy for present-day living.

In Loewald's (1960) words:

> The transference neurosis, in the technical sense of the establishment and resolution of it in the analytic process, is due to the blood of recognition which the patient's unconscious is given to taste—so that the old ghosts may reawaken to life.[1] Those who know ghosts tell us that they long to be released from their ghost-life and led to rest as ancestors. As ancestors they live forth in the present generation, while as ghosts they are compelled to haunt the present generation with their shadow-life. Transference is pathological in so far as the unconscious is a crowd of ghosts, and this is the beginning of the transference neurosis in analysis: ghosts of the unconscious, imprisoned by defences but haunting the patient in the dark of his defences and symptoms, are allowed to taste blood, are let loose. In the daylight of analysis the ghosts of the unconscious are laid and led to rest as ancestors whose power is taken over and transformed into the newer intensity of present life, of the secondary process and contemporary objects.
>
> (p. 29)

Loewald's ghost metaphor arises out of the traditional psychoanalytic emphasis on the dynamic, or motivated, unconscious (as distinguished from what can be called the descriptive unconscious, which would include everything not in awareness at a particular moment). Loewald's ghosts are thus the products of *repression,* along with various other ego defenses that have been employed to protect against early psychic conflict. In this model of mind, an individual's unconscious ghosts—the conflictual internalized object relationships of childhood—are understood to be the primary fashioners of personality structure and the organizers of psychic life.

For many analysts today, psychic life is conceived as being primarily organized as multiple self states arising from the *dissociation* of experience that cannot be metabolized (e.g., Benjamin 2010; Bromberg 2003, 2006,

2011; Davies 1998; Davies and Frawley 1994; Stern 2009). Dissociation is understood as an automatic, biologically based self-protective mechanism rather than as a motivated defense. In this conception, it is in a separate self state or states that aspects of unmetabolizable experience and unintegratable objects reside. In the most extreme situation—dissociative identity disorder—the sequelae of traumatic experiences are split off into entirely separate, multiple personalities.

In my opinion, the different defensive/protective mechanisms emphasized in these two conceptions of mind need not be considered opposed to each other. Dissociation—which may be a motivated defense as well as an automatic protective mechanism—-and repression interact in complex ways. The psychological issues we work with are multiply determined, layered mixtures of both (see also Smith 2000) even when it comes to trauma. Trauma is best understood not simply as an environmental event, but as a particular interaction between a complex psyche and the environment. Psychic trauma exists on a continuum from "small-t" trauma to the more extreme kinds of "capital-T" Trauma. The dissociative mechanisms employed to cope with such experiences also range in their severity and in their impact on personality and functioning (Laub and Auerhahn 1993), and not all necessarily lead to "multiple" self states.

Further, all of the developmental challenges and psychic conflicts of childhood will be experienced as more or less traumatic depending on the environmental context. And every trauma, whether in early childhood or contemporary, capital-T or small-t, will be personally elaborated and colored, organized and reorganized, by ongoing unconscious fantasies, meanings, and conflicting affects. There is always an admixture of repressive and dissociative processes, with the balance perhaps determined by the degree to which the ego or coherence of the self feels overwhelmed and threatened with psychic annihilation.

The above notwithstanding, the differences between these two defensive/protective mechanisms, repression and dissociation, lend themselves to different metaphors for capturing the patient's experience. While Loewald's (1960) metaphor of a ghost aptly captures the recurrent haunting that one experiences from a repressed, conflictual early object relationship, I suggest that the metaphor of a vampire best captures the overwhelming kind of terror and menace that one may experience from a dissociated trauma. In this chapter, I will draw the categories of repressed ghosts and dissociated vampires as if they were pure forms because these metaphors provide, for both the patient and the treating clinician, vivid, experience-near imagery for each of these psychic experiences.

I will begin with descriptions of how ghosts and vampires are depicted in folklore and the ways they are experienced in analytic treatment. I will give greater focus to the vampire metaphor as it has been less extensively explored. I will then describe the enacted dimension of analytic process, the arena of treatment in which all demons are inevitably revivified, "recognized," and ultimately laid to rest as ancestors. I will then present an extensive clinical illustration of a dissociated vampire.

Ghosts and vampires in folklore and analytic treatment

In literature and film, ghosts and vampires are depicted differently. Ghosts haunt; vampires assault. Vampires wreak anguished bodily harm and even death. In everyday life, we have all experienced the hauntings of repressed ghosts—conflictual issues from childhood, now repressed, can generate contemporary feelings of diffuse anxiety, nagging guilt, and unaccounted-for dysphoria. An overwhelming trauma that had to be dissociated, however, generally feels more like some external, *not-me* entity or force— more like an alien, menacing vampire that must be kept, at all cost, at great psychic distance. To be in any kind of contact with a dissociated trauma is to consort with something believed to be lethal. It is to experience more than the disquieting affects of one's repressed ghosts; it is to feel the threat of extreme psychic pain, even psychic annihilation.

In psychoanalytic treatment, traces of an individual's ghosts—the now-repressed conflictual object relationships of childhood populating the dynamic unconscious—may regularly be detected in day-to-day work. They are in disguise as symptoms and other compromise formations, woven into and hidden in ego-syntonic character traits. Patients generally try to describe, to put into words, the emotional haunting they feel, and the analyst's clarifications and interpretive comments about the ghost at hand will make increasing sense to the patient and gradually begin to have an ameliorative effect.

In contrast, as clinical experience shows, a traumatic experience that has never been formulated is often inaccessible and unsymbolizable in treatment for many years. The patient has neither the capacity to tolerate it nor the words to talk about it. Even if the analyst has some knowledge or sense that there is trauma in the patient's history, his or her words, particularly in the early phase of treatment, will either be rebuffed or will (re)traumatize the patient. Like the vampire that cannot survive in the sun, a dissociated trauma cannot exist initially in the "daylight of analysis." Enshrouded in the darkness of its own separate, alien self state, it lurks at the edges of the patient's consciousness and on the fringes of the treatment, nameless yet deeply terrifying, for a long time.

In Loewald's (1960) metaphor, ghosts do not wish to continue to live in the shadows as defensively unintegrated parts of one's personality who can only distort and warp present-day life. They long to be freed and to take their rightful place as integrated ancestral components of one's personality, to become useful influences in contemporary life. Proust (1913–1927) described this process as follows:

> When we have passed a certain age, the soul of the child that we were and the souls of the dead from whom we sprang come and shower upon us their riches and their spells, asking to be allowed to contribute to the new emotions which we feel and in which, erasing their former image, we recast them in an original creation.
>
> (p. 73)

Thus, when a repressed ghost enters the treatment process, it bears a gift for the patient, a gift the analyst helps liberate. In contrast, aspects of a traumatic experience or a traumatic relationship that remain unformulated—dissociated rather than repressed—are generally experienced as *not-me,* as terrifying entities to be avoided at all costs, rather than as something that may potentially bear a gift. Like the vampire in its crypt that is neither living nor dead, a dissociated trauma tends to remain in its own "undead" sector of the self—unformulated, unprocessed. It does not seek the blood of emotional recognition; it seeks the emotional lifeblood of its victim, steadily depleting his or her sense of self in order to sustain its own dissociated, malevolent existence.

Specific traumas and the vampire metaphor

While every trauma is unique to the particular patient's history and psyche, there are some specific categories of trauma that have attracted the attention of psychoanalytic clinicians, researchers and writers. I will here focus on three particular traumas—unmourned object loss, sexual abuse, and trauma that has been intergenerationally transmitted—to illustrate how the vampire metaphor captures the well-known self and object experience of these patients.

Unmourned object loss

The process of mourning is a most difficult one, a process that even under the most favorable conditions is perhaps never fully completed. In the best circumstances, the lost object is eventually laid to rest as an ancestral part of one's personality. If the loss has been traumatic, however, the individual may deny and dissociate the trauma, even while accepting the reality of the death in a more rational sector of the self. For such an individual, the lost object has not truly died.[2]

The vampire metaphor captures several aspects of this experience. In legend and myth, a vampire was considered to be a person who had died, suddenly and unexpectedly, "before his or her time," but who nevertheless retains its original corporeal existence in the real world for generations. Similarly, an unmourned love object retains its pre-death psychic existence in the dissociated sector of the personality—never aging, frozen in time. Gottlieb (1994) and Yassa and Smith (2000) have shown that the relationship with the unmourned object may actually come to be represented in analytic treatment through vampire dreams, images and fantasies. Not only does the shadow of the object fall upon the ego (Freud 1917), but the actual lost, unmourned loved one—now unlost and undead—returns at night, in dreams and nightmares, appearing just the same as he or she did before death, no matter how many years have passed.

But although the person and the lost love object are reunited in this way, the reunion is a parasitic one, devoid of true object relatedness. The vampire—the dissociated embodiment of unmourned loss, imbued with the darkness of unresolved pain and anger—drains the individual of vitality, ultimately turning the victim into a kind of undead creature as well, one who is unable to be fully involved in contemporary relationships.

The sexual abuser

As portrayed in literature and film, vampires are potent sexual figures, dripping with insatiable need and hunger, full of sexual and aggressive power. A vampire seduces, mesmerizes, excites and penetrates. It ravishes and violates. Unable to offer resistance, its victim becomes steadily weakened and ill. In this respect, the vampire metaphor personifies the sexual predator and abuser who is dependent on the passive cooperation of its victim in order to survive, and to whom the victim, helpless in the face of its power, continues to be in thrall.

When the victim is a child and the abuser is a parent or caregiver on whom the child is totally dependent, the child's maturational needs for attachment and for the development of a coherent sense of self, unrecognized and unmet by the abuser, come to be experienced as unacceptable. As these unmet needs become ever more infected with continuing abuse and entwined with the wishes and fantasies of the child's evolving sexuality and aggression, the child's experience of him/herself inevitably becomes infused with abusing and sadomasochistic characteristics.

Experienced as dangerous, even life-threatening, these aggressive aspects of the child's identity need to be disavowed and relocated in a split-off self state (what Faimberg [2005] and Fonagy [2008] call an *alien self*) and/or externalized and projected onto others. The dissociated "vampire self" (or alter, should the traumatic abuse result in a dissociative identity disorder), and those in the external world who are targets of the projections, become repositories of the insatiable aggressive/sexual hunger, leaving the individual depleted and drained of healthy object relational capacity.

Intergenerational transmission

The effects of any kind of massive trauma do not merely remain dissociated in the victim. In psychoanalytic treatment, we are witness to patients for whom the dissociated trauma of an earlier generation has been transmitted to them. The subject of intergenerational transmission of trauma has generated a considerable amount of psychoanalytic literature. The vampire metaphor captures this kind of transmission vividly; in most renditions of the legend, the vampire's bite does not kill but rather serves to transmit its "illness"—to create a new vampire that lives on to prey on the next generation.

From various perspectives, such writers as Laub and Auerhahn (1993), Grand (2000), Faimberg (2005) and Fromm (2012) describe an array of identificatory, defensive and object relational mechanisms involved in this transmission process. The unformulated and dissociated affects and images of the original victim's traumatic experience may be unconsciously identified with by his or her child, and/or intruded into the child by the parent.[3] The child may also identify with the parent's traumatizing modes of relating, which are a product of the parent's own unconscious identification with his or her aggressor. All these processes will then eventuate in the original survivor's trauma becoming an alive but unformulated part of the child's psyche, and then, in similar fashion, being transmitted to the third-generation survivor.

*

Thus far, I have made sharp distinctions between repression and dissociation through the metaphors of ghosts and vampires. As noted earlier, there is more overlap and complexity than these discrete categories convey. Not every unrepresented or dissociated state will be experienced as a menacing vampire, just as there is a sense in which all repressed wishes and conflicts are experienced as alien. Nevertheless, the addition of the dissociated vampire metaphor to Loewald's repressed ghost metaphor usefully captures aspects of the experience of patients who suffer from the effects of various kinds of overwhelming, (capital-T) Trauma—in particular, survivors and the offspring of survivors of childhood sexual abuse, unmournable early object loss and genocide.

Regardless of whether the patient's demon is repressed, dissociated or some mixture of the two, it will inevitably return to life in the treatment's enacted realm. The further toward the "repressed ghosts" end of the continuum one's demon is, the more work can be done in the verbal dimension of the treatment, although its revivification will inevitably be taking place, simultaneously and without awareness, in the enacted dimension as well, which will become a crucial part of the effectiveness of the working though process. The further a trauma is toward the "dissociated vampire" end of the continuum, the more it can only be accessed as it becomes revivified in the enacted dimension. It is to this dimension of the treatment process that I will now turn.

The enacted dimension: the scene of the action

In a successful analytic treatment, a patient's ghosts and vampires—experiences that have been relegated to the repressed unconscious or expelled into the netherworld of the dissociated undead—will be laid to rest as ancestors. To achieve this outcome, the undead must first return to life in the here and now of the analytic dyad—in a form that is less traumatic and more benign, in a form that makes them accessible to analytic treatment. In this section, I will define what I call the *enacted dimension of analytic process* in order to explore how both ghosts and vampires—while experienced differently—ultimately make their appearance enactively in the transference-countertransference matrix.

As I will describe presently, the enacted dimension is a naturally occurring, descriptive part of analytic *process*, not a prescriptive part of analytic technique. Thus I will not be addressing particular strategies or different approaches to treating "ghosts" or "vampires." Rather, I will focus on an *ongoing unconscious arena* of analytic process—present regardless of the analyst's technical approach—in which both the repressed as well as the dissociated make their appearance.

I will begin by reviewing and expanding on the process inherent in Loewald's (1960) original metaphor of transforming ghosts into ancestors, a forerunner of the enacted dimension. Loewald considered the transference neurosis the arena in which repressed ghosts taste the blood of recognition and come to life. He understood the transference neurosis as evolving within an interactive, transference-countertransference field—in the interaction between the analyst's and patient's different roles and ways of psychic functioning in the analytic undertaking:

> In the development of the psychic apparatus the secondary process, preconscious organization, is the manifestation and result of interaction between a more primitively organized psychic apparatus and the secondary process activity of the environment; through such interaction the unconscious gains higher organization. Such ego-development, arrested or distorted in neurosis, is resumed in analysis. The analyst helps to revive the repressed unconscious of the patient by his recognition of it; through interpretation of transference and resistance, through the recovery of memories and through reconstruction, the patient's unconscious activity is led into preconscious organization. The analyst, in the analytic situation, offers himself to the patient as a contemporary object. As such he revives the ghosts of the unconscious for the patient by fostering the transference neurosis, which comes about in the same way in which the dream comes about: through the mutual attraction of unconscious and "recent," "day residue" elements. Dream interpretation and interpretation of transference

have this function in common: they both attempt to re-establish the lost connexions, the buried interplay, between the unconscious and the preconscious.

(pp. 29–30)

Loewald is here primarily describing the *verbally* symbolic aspects of what transpires in day-to-day work within the interactive transference-countertransference field. In Loewald's metaphor, the repressed ghosts of the patient's past are genuinely welcomed into the treatment as transference, and the patient comes to gradually recognize them through the juxtaposed experience of the analyst as both an old (ghost) object and a contemporary object. The ongoing processes of interpretation, recovery of memories, reconstruction and working through enable repressed ghosts to then finally be internalized as psychic structure, as integrated aspects of one's personality.

In later papers, as I shall describe in what follows, Loewald foreshadowed contemporary interest in enacted processes—early *nonverbal* forms of symbolization and communication—in such concepts as *language action* and *enactive memory,* reflecting a prescient understanding that the transference neurosis and the transference-countertransference field consist of more than what is communicated in representational language.

This additional facet of the transference-countertransference field is its *enacted dimension*. It is in this unconsciously evolving realm of analytic process that patients have the vivid experience that their demons—both ghosts and vampires—have returned to life in the here-and-now reality of the treatment relationship. The enacted dimension is the continuous, *interpsychic*[4] dimension of all treatment relationships that evolves, without the awareness or intent of either party, side by side and interwoven with the day-to-day content of clinical work—the more familiar, verbally symbolized dimension of the treatment. In the enacted dimension, the patient inevitably induces the analyst to play a part in, and thereby to *actualize*, an unconscious object relationship or traumatic experience.[5] The patient's ghost or the patient's vampire tastes the blood of recognition in the *analyst's* unconscious. (I will illustrate this idea in the case presentation that follows.)

As this dimension of the transference-countertransference matrix evolves, a new edition—a new treatment version—of the early relationship or trauma is created (what Poland [1992], citing the passage from Proust that I quoted earlier, calls an *original creation*) that feels immediate, real, and effectively alive. In this new edition, the past is not just remembered, it is *re-lived*—but in an attenuated, less traumatic form, making possible the ultimate transformation from ghosts into ancestors.

Loewald alludes to this heightened sense of reality, a central feature of the enacted dimension, in the quotation cited earlier, when he likens the transference neurosis to a dream. Dreams feel real. In a dream, repressed ghosts and dissociated vampires use visual and auditory images to provide them with vivid, experientially real expression. In the enacted dimension, they use action (both motor action and verbal action) to provide them with the same kind of vivid, experientially real expression. When this "two-party," waking dream[6] becomes conscious, it forms the basis for experientially based interpretive work in the verbally symbolic dimension of the treatment, creating a unique kind of *experiential insight*—insight about a past that is palpably alive in the present, the kind of insight that produces meaningful psychoanalytic change. The patient's ongoing experience of the oscillation between both dimensions of the treatment—between the realm of reawakened ghosts and vampires and the realm of the analyst as a contemporary object—provides him or her with the opportunity to reopen early paths of development, within which new ways of relating to one's objects and to oneself can be discovered.

The enactive, performative, living quality of what is experienced in the enacted dimension of analytic process is also highlighted by Loewald in later papers (1971, 1975, 1976), in which he discusses the difference between *representational memory* and *enactive memory* (*repetition by action*), and likens the transference neurosis to a dramatic play that takes place in the process between patient and analyst: "Viewed as a dramatic play, the transference neurosis is a fantasy creation woven from memories and imaginative elaborations of present actuality, the present actuality being the psychoanalytic situation, the relationship of patient and analyst" (1975, p. 279).

In this dramatic play—what I have called the play within the play (Katz 2014)—communicative language is increasingly transformed into action forms of language, what Loewald (1975) calls *language action*,[7] which is the major vehicle for the actualization processes that take place in the enacted dimension of the treatment:

> In the course of the psychoanalytic process, narrative is drawn into the context of transference dramatization, into the force-field of re-enactment. Whether in the form of free association or of more

consciously, logically controlled trains of thought, narrative in psychoanalysis is increasingly being revealed in its character as language action, as symbolic action, and in particular as language action within the transference force-field. The emphasis, in regard to content and emotional tone of the communications through narrative, shifts more and more to their relevance as transference repetitions and transference actions in the psychoanalytic situation. One might express this by saying that we take the patient less and less as speaking merely about himself, about his experiences and memories, and more and more as symbolizing action in speech, as speaking from the depth of his memories, which regain life and poignancy by the impetus and urgency of re-experience in the present of the analytic situation.

(pp. 293–294)

Thus, despite the talking cure's historical emphasis on verbal symbolization, we now appreciate the extent to which the core experiences of one's life are remembered and represented in treatment not only in the verbal sphere, but also—inescapably, and sometimes exclusively—in the enactive sphere. Repressed ghosts and dissociated vampires return to life in analytic treatment on the sensorimotor, affect/somatic level, and also through various *action* forms of *language*.[8] All experiences and relationships that could not be symbolized verbally at the time of their occurrence—either because they were preverbal and had no words, or because they were too traumatic and conflicted—return to life in the treatment's enacted dimension.

To further "enliven" these ideas, I will turn next to the case of Ann. This treatment, which I supervised, illustrates the following:

(a) how the traumatic experience of the Holocaust, which could not be processed by the original victims, the patient's grandparents, had been transmitted across three generations of survivors to the patient;
(b) the relevance of the vampire metaphor—which the patient introduced herself—to her experience of the dissociated traumatic affects and images that exerted enormous power and control over her life; and
(c) the particular defensive arrangement that the patient and her mother had created and perpetuated in their relationship to protect both of them from knowledge of the trauma—which, from the beginning of the treatment and for an extended period, was re-created, without awareness, in the enacted dimension of the analytic dyad. As their

reenactment gradually became recognized and available for verbal symbolization, the patient's menacing, vampiric trauma could finally be consciously known.

The intergenerational transmission of a Holocaust vampire: the case of Ann[9]

Ann was a talented, 32-year-old artist. She came to treatment saying she experienced "complicated emotional processes" that she wanted to understand: "My experience is sometimes like I have many parts to myself that I need to put together . . . I want to reach a better integration."

Ann also suffered from somatic symptoms, particularly stomach problems, and was tormented by eating rituals. She described difficulties forming close relationships, especially romantic relationships with men. She managed to avoid serious relationships by moving every two to three years to a different city or even a different country, unable to put down roots anywhere and create her own home. She said: "I am like a street cat that has no home and gets along everywhere . . . or maybe I am more like a turtle whose home is always with him . . . I need only a small suitcase in which I can easily pack myself—several clothes, some books, my art creations—and here I am, on my way again."

From the beginning of the analysis, Ann exhibited frequent states of traumatic affect—severe anxiety, panic states, acute mortification—that she could not name or process. On her way to one of her first analytic sessions, she had an intense anxiety attack when her subway train became stuck in a tunnel. In the closed and crowded train car, she felt a claustrophobic panic as she breathed in the sour air surrounding her. In any given session, she might be flooded by diffuse and contentless anxiety, and then in the very next session be emotionally numb and talk about an interaction or event that appeared related to, but which she did not and could not connect to, the anxiety of the previous session. For Ann, there were affect states without content, images without feelings, horror without a story.

The nature of these dissociated states and these traumatic affects and images became understandable only after Ann learned—for the first time almost a year into the treatment—of her family's Holocaust experience. Ann was a third-generation Holocaust survivor. Much of her mother's extended family were annihilated; in particular, both of Ann's maternal grandparents lost both their parents. Much of her father's extended family were expelled from their homes and communities, forced to wander from country to country.

The emotional experiences and images of these devastating traumas were transmitted from generation to generation—from her grandparents, to her parents, to Ann—without ever being put into words. There was an unspoken prohibition against verbalizing anything about the Holocaust. She and her mother never talked about their family's history—nor, for that matter, about any emotionally charged aspect of their relationship. These were communicated either nonverbally or through a secret language that they had always had with each other, what Ann called their "code." For example, comments about the weather were understood by both mother and daughter as comments about the atmosphere between them; comments about physical ailments were a communication about the emotional pain that one was causing the other.

Ann's idiosyncratic relationship with her mother was captured in a dream she had during the first year of analysis about a chocolate bar, still in its wrapper, but which was separated into two halves within it. Ann and her mother were separate and attached at the same time. They were physically and geographically separate, and in many ways psychologically differentiated, yet they were emotionally bound together in a symbiotic wrapper within which they remained safe from the unspeakable horrors of the Holocaust—which were, simultaneously, wordlessly transmitted. The two pieces of the chocolate bar also captured the way that the Holocaust trauma was sequestered in an entirely separate sector of Ann's personality, dissociated from her otherwise intact symbolizing capacities.

It was the extended work on this and related dreams, images, and artistic creations that finally led Ann, late in the first year of analysis, to talk to her mother about what it was that they were always not talking about, always avoiding, always terrified about. This eventuated in her finally learning of her grandparents' Holocaust trauma—the dissociated vampire that had menaced three generations of her family.

Despite the fact that Ann had no conscious knowledge of her family history while growing up, that history had nevertheless registered in her body and in her psyche, and came to affect virtually every aspect of her functioning and daily life. Encoded on the sensorimotor level, the trauma found expression in Ann's unmetabolized affect states, somatic symptoms, and eating rituals. Relationally, it found expression in her propensity to live her life as a "wandering Jew:" her near-compulsive need to move to a different country every couple of years (as her paternal grandfather was forced to do). In fact, Ann avoided meaningful relationships by moving from place to place, in effect trying to stay one step ahead of her depressed, dissociated vampire who was always threatening to find her.

The split-off experience of her family's Holocaust trauma was also represented and expressed—and without any conscious awareness—in her paintings and other artistic creations. Many of the paintings depicted leaving, moving, and searching for a home that could never be reached. Moreover, tidal waves and destruction were frequent dream images.

The most important way that dissociated aspects of the trauma found expression and representation in Ann's treatment was in its enacted dimension. As I will illustrate, what found symbolic actualization in the transference-countertransference matrix was not only the dissociated affects and existential anxieties of the Holocaust, but also the nonverbal and unacknowledged arrangement with her mother—the chocolate bar relationship—that maintained the dissociation.

Ann's vampire story

Before turning to the treatment's enacted dimension in detail, I will describe the nineteenth-century vampire story that Ann related in the second year of treatment, which occupied the analytic work for several weeks.[10] As noted, through the work on the chocolate bar metaphor, Ann was becoming more open to exploring what the idiosyncratic ways of relating that she and her mother had developed were protecting them from—what she called their "dangerously emotional relationship."

The vampire story she related—without fully knowing what she was trying to communicate—was about women vampires who formed intimate, erotic bonds with their female victims.[11] The narrator was a young girl who had become a victim of a beautiful and seductive woman vampire. Gradually and patiently, the vampire tempted her into a love relationship and would secretly bite her on her breast while she was asleep. Every bite made the girl more ill, as through this process the illness of the vampire was transmitted to her. The illness was a kind of depression, Ann stated, as the girl became drained of all her vitality. The girl was about to die and turn into a vampire herself, extending the line of vampires into a new generation, but she was saved at the last moment by her father.

Ann's vampire story captures her experience of the "dangerously emotional relationship" with her mother and the way the Holocaust trauma was transmitted to her. For Ann, the vampire's "illness," the unspeakable traumatic affects and images of the Holocaust, was passed on through nonverbal forms of oral transmission—through what she incorporated along with mother's milk (symbolically, in reversed form, the vampire bite was on the breast) and through the intimacy of more adult forms of love and attachment. For Ann, it became dangerous to love. Love was poisonous and deadly.

Ann commented while talking about the vampire story: "When I get close to another person, I feel as if an open channel is formed between us and things are transmitted between us without my being able to choose what to take in and what to leave out." She became afraid, she said, that she would absorb bad things that belonged to the other person, and that good things would be drained out of her. That was how it was with her mother, who transmitted to Ann her own depression, inner deadness, and unmourned trauma, all of which were still sapping Ann of her vitality. Indeed, in the treatment's early months, following difficult emotional interactions with her mother, she had sometimes talked about not feeling well physically, feeling that perhaps some "weird virus" had intruded into her. She would then go on a severe fasting diet to purge and cleanse herself.

Ann's vampire story not only illustrates how massive, dissociated trauma is passed on nonverbally from one generation to the next; it also suggests how the dissociative pattern in the recipient may be elaborated and reworked across different levels of development. In Ann's story, the trauma is transmitted not only on the oral incorporative level, through maternal merger, but also through erotic/sexual interaction with the female vampire. In addition, the story has a triadic cast with the introduction of the father as a third who saves the daughter not only from preoedipal attachment to the mother, but also from later erotic enmeshment with her.

One can also see in this story Ann's defensive identification with her dissociated vampire. In the way she lived her life, Ann *became* the vampire. She roamed restlessly from country to country, contaminating relationship after relationship, unable to find peace and rest. In the treatment, experiencing herself as an already contaminated incipient vampire, she feared that any closeness with her (female) analyst would transfer her illness/virus to the analyst and destroy the treatment.

As I will now elaborate, before Ann could consciously know of and integrate the dissociated emotional experience of her grandparents' Holocaust trauma into her personality structure, a new version of defensive arrangement by which she and her mother maintained the trauma in a dissociated state had to become a living part of the transference-countertransference matrix.

The enacted dimension of Ann's analysis

From the treatment's inception, Ann and her analyst had been, without awareness, re-creating the highly idiosyncratic ways of relating developed by mother and daughter—the chocolate bar relationship. This enacted aspect of the analytic relationship formed its continuous backdrop, but it only became conscious and understandable in retrospect. For long and intense periods, patient and analyst literally felt enveloped in that chocolate bar wrapper—secretly attached and secretly separate—neither able to talk about substantial areas of their experience together. As Ann and her mother had long done, her analyst found herself speaking with Ann in code—not talking about the real thing or talking in displaced arenas, both of them fully knowing, but never acknowledging, what they were really talking about. They walked on eggshells with each other—Ann fearful that any expression of her more differentiated self would destroy her analyst, and her analyst fearful that any intervention, or any non-intervention, would destroy the treatment.

So sealed in their wrapper were they that, at moments, the analyst actually felt what she presumed was *Ann's* unformulated, inchoate terror, yet could not be sure from whom or from where this experience originated; there was "no membrane," to use Ann's expression. They were reliving the original "emotionally dangerous" relationship that neither wanted to be in, but from which neither could leave.

The analyst reported later that, during this period, she often felt a strong resistance to sharing the clinical process in supervision with me. In addition to being the father/third who could save them, I as the supervisor had become the lurking, dangerous vampire that she and Ann, wrapped together in their wrapper, had to avoid. And even as the material about the Holocaust finally began to emerge, Ann's analyst found herself feeling that discussion with Ann of any experience of attachment and loss—particularly as manifested in the analytic relationship around weekends and other analytic breaks—was inadmissible, a dangerous and forbidden subject in the analysis, the same taboo under which three generations of Holocaust survivors had suffered. In other words, without being fully conscious of it, both feared that any breach in the mutual dissociation inherent in their arrangement would allow the traumatic, vampiric experiences into the room before they were ready to deal with them.

This re-creation in the transference-countertransference was abruptly shattered one day when the analyst, without conscious planning, suddenly found herself putting into words for Ann—in one lengthy, powerful intervention, and with what was for her an atypical degree of intensity and comprehensiveness—everything she had actually come to understand about her patient over a period of time, but what from her position within the transference-countertransference wrapper she had not previously been able to utter. With more emotion and less of her usual caution, she spoke to Ann about Ann's Holocaust history, about the trauma her grandparents and mother had suffered. She spoke to her about the resulting chocolate bar relationship with her mother that protected them from the trauma, but that also made Ann terrified to take the risk of feeling attached to anyone. And the analyst described in detail how all this had been re-created between them in the treatment.

The analyst worried about the possible effects of her unusual intervention, but she also felt freed, and the treatment suddenly felt more alive. It was as if the allied forces had liberated the camps—or, to return to this chapter's theme, it was as if a wooden stake had been suddenly driven into the heart of the vampire—and a new world became visible and possible. Ann, too, seemed relieved. As the session ended and she rose from the couch, she looked her analyst in the eye more directly than was typical, smiled, and said thank you.

I would like to point out that the analyst's unplanned intervention was *part and parcel* of the enacted process: A response to what was likely Ann's unconscious communications that, in the context of the greater safety of treatment, she was ready—and the analyst was ready (discussed in the next section)—to emerge from the maternal transference-countertransference wrapper that they had been bound together in for nearly a year and a half. This allowed Ann to begin the process of bearing witness to and *integrating*—rather than dissociating—this aspect of her psychic heritage and of coming to terms with it as best she might. Through this lengthy enacted process, Ann had the opportunity to convert what had been passively endured in childhood into something that she actively (even if unconsciously) intended, and that she could now begin to actively master.

Once the dissociated Holocaust vampire could find conscious verbal representation in the treatment, Ann began to examine the many ways it had impacted her personality, her artistic productions, and her relationship choices. As the analysis progressed, the many layers of psychic meaning and defense that subsequently became attached to the Holocaust trauma could be gradually worked through. This process also enabled issues that had been obscured by the trauma—other aspects of her relationship with her mother, and her many-faceted relationship with her father—to take their place in the analytic work.

The analyst's ghosts and vampires

As I have described, the enacted dimension evolves through the interpsychic interpenetration that transpires within the transference-countertransference matrix. An enacted process is as unique as each patient-analyst dyad; it is a unique product of both psyches. Thus, in the enacted dimension, the patient's repressed ghosts and dissociated vampires taste the blood of recognition in the unconscious and unformulated areas of the *analyst's* personality that have been activated by those of the patient.

During the same period that Ann was learning of her Holocaust history, Ann's analyst discovered that, unbeknownst to her, she herself had a Holocaust history that her family had never discussed. While aware of some general similarities between her patient's object relationship patterns and anxiety states and her own, after learning of Ann's Holocaust history, the analyst began to realize that there were similarities in their family dynamics—in particular, an aversion to discussing emotional matters, frequent charged silences, and separation and separateness issues. She began to wonder about her own familial history. She knew that her parents had emigrated from Europe shortly before the Second World War, but realized that she had no idea whether there had been members of her extended family who might have stayed behind and what might have happened to them. She discovered that several relatives, on both sides of her family, had indeed remained and were lost in the Holocaust. Unbeknownst to her, and without conscious intent on their part, her parents had bequeathed to her their own dissociated Holocaust vampire.

While it had remained internally unformulated during the early portion of her treatment of Ann, the analyst's dissociated vampire had perhaps been "recognized" by Ann's, enabling Ann to induce her analyst to join her in the chocolate bar wrapper. Both patient and analyst had an initial investment in keeping their vampires in the dark, as neither was ready to have them emerge into the sunlight. As their secret separateness within their protective wrapper gradually strengthened, and as each began to learn of her Holocaust vampire, the analyst suddenly found herself making the long, unplanned interpretation described earlier.

The analyst's ability to face her own dissociated traumatic affects, in conjunction with the beginning readiness in Ann to face hers, allowed the analyst to make interpretive connections for her patient that were now based on and firmly rooted in the live, experiential immediacy of their analytic relationship. Patient and analyst could begin to emerge from the protection of their wrapper, and Ann could now begin—in the "daylight of analysis" (Loewald 1960, p. 29)—to lead and lay her dissociated vampire to rest.

Summary and conclusion

Starting with Loewald's (1960) metaphor of transforming the ghosts of the past into ancestors, which usefully captures the recurrent haunting that one experiences from repressed, conflictual early object relationships, I have offered the metaphor of the *dissociated vampire* to portray the particular kind of danger and terror one experiences from an overwhelming trauma that could not be formulated or processed. I then described how ghosts and vampires are depicted in legend, literature, and film, and how they are experienced in the treatment process. While the sharp distinction made between repression and dissociation is admittedly an oversimplification, the vampire metaphor illuminates and captures, with experience-near imagery, the experience of many patients who suffer from the effects of various kinds of overwhelming trauma—in particular, survivors and the offspring of survivors of childhood sexual abuse, unmournable early object loss, and genocide.

I have then gone on to describe the enacted dimension of psychoanalytic process and its origins in Loewald's seminal writings. The enacted dimension is the continuous, interpsychic dimension of all treatment relationships that evolves, without the awareness or intent of either analyst or patient, side-by-side and interwoven with the day-to-day content of clinical work. In this enacted dimension—the play within the play (Katz 2014) the patient inevitably induces the analyst into playing a part in, and thereby actualizing, an unconscious object relationship or traumatic experience. It is in this continuously evolving dimension of the treatment process that the patient's ghosts or vampires come to life in the treatment relationship, providing the opportunity for their being verbally symbolized and laid to rest.

Lastly I have included an extensive clinical illustration of the major themes of the paper:

(a) the relevance of the vampire metaphor to the patient's experience of a dissociated trauma that had been transmitted to her across three generations of Holocaust survivors;
(b) the nature of the very particular defensive arrangement that had been created between herself and her mother to protect both of them from knowledge and experience of the trauma; and
(c) the way in which this relationshop was re-created in the enacted dimension of the analytic dyad, enabling this menacing "vampire" to fully enter the treatment and finally be lain to rest.

Coda

Analysts usefully employ many different metaphors—ghosts, vampires, and various species of the undead—to depict what plagues and possesses our patients and to conceptualize the dynamics of each patient's experience. Ultimately, analytic work involves the process of allowing the undead to return to life in the treatment's enacted dimension, and transforming psychic demons into ancestors and traumatic experiences into memories.

Notes

1 Loewald borrowed this metaphor from Freud (1900), who used it to describe the indestructible nature of the Unconscious. Freud was referencing the "ghosts in the underworld of the Odyssey—ghosts which awoke to new life as soon as they tasted blood" (p. 553n).
2 See Frankiel (1994) for clinical examples.
3 See Faimberg's (2005) ideas about intrusion and appropriation.
4 I use the term *interpsychic interaction* (see Bolognini 2011; Loewald 1970) to refer to the preconscious/unconscious communication that evolves between the two psyches in the analytic situation. It is thus not strictly inter-*personal* (the more *conscious* interactions between two *people*, as opposed to two *psyches*), and it is not strictly

intra-psychic, as two intrapsychic psyches are involved. *Interpsychic communication* creates the realm in which unconscious dynamics, situated independently in patient and analyst, are communicated, take shape, and find expression in overt action or through the ordinary verbal interaction of the analytic encounter.

5 See also Sandler's (1976) concept of *role responsiveness,* Boesky's (1990) ideas about *unconsciously negotiated resistance,* and Levenson's (1972) description of *transformation and resisting transformation.*
6 See also Loewald's (1975) ideas, discussed later in this paper, about psychoanalysis as a *dramatic play,* Kern's (1987) formulation of the transference neurosis as a *waking dream* or a *psychodrama for two,* and Cassorla's (2005, 2013) concepts, from a Bionian perspective, of the *consulting room theatre* and the *dream for two.*
7 See also Busch's (1989) concept of *action thoughts* and Levenson's (1983) use of the term *language act.* For contemporary appreciations of Loewald's theories of the interplay between enactive and representational forms of language, experience, and memory, in both human development and therapeutic process, see Singer and Conway (2011) and Vivona (2003, 2006, 2009).
8 Here we might think of what Dowling (1982) calls *motor recognitions,* of Bromberg's (2003) *affective memories,* and of Busch's (1989) *memories in action.*
9 I thank Michal Talby-Abarbanel and her patient "Ann" for their permission to publish this treatment material.
10 Though it was never cited by Ann, the story was likely *Carmilla* (Le Fanu 1871), a Gothic novella about a female vampire. *Carmilla* pre-dates *Dracula* (Stoker 1897), which it greatly influenced, by some years, and has been adapted in several film versions.
11 While vampires in popular American culture, which are based on Western European vampire myths, are generally male, in earlier, Eastern vampire myths the vampire was almost always female (Wilson 2000).

This chapter first appeared as 'Repressed ghosts and dissociated vampires in the enacted dimension of psychoanalytic treatment' in *The Psychoanalytic Quarterly*, Volume 84, Issue 2, pages 389–414, April 2015. Reprinted by permission of the journal and John Wiley and Sons, Inc.

Bibliography

Benjamin, J. (2010). Where's the gap and what's the difference? The relational view of intersubjectivity, multiple selves, and enactments. *Contemp. Psychoanal.*, 46:112–119.
Boesky, D. (1990). The psychoanalytic process and its components. *Psychoanal. Q.*, 59:550–584.
Bolognini, S. (2011). *Secret Passages: The Theory and Technique of Interpsychic Relations,* trans. G. Atkinson. London: Routledge.
Bromberg, P. M. (2003). One need not be a house to be haunted: on enactment, dissociation, and the dread of "not-me": a case study. *Psychoanal. Dialogues*, 13:689–709.
——— (2006). *Awakening the Dreamer: Clinical Journeys.* Hillsdale, NJ: The Analytic Press.
——— (2011). *The Shadow of the Tsunami and the Growth of the Relational Mind.* New York, NY: Routledge.
Busch, F. (1989). The compulsion to repeat in action: a developmental perspective. *Int. J. Psychoanal.*, 70:535–544.
Cassorla, R. M. (2005). From bastion to enactment: the "non-dream" in the theatre of analysis. *Int. J. Psychoanal.*, 86:699–719.

——— (2013). When the analyst becomes stupid: an attempt to understand enactment using Bion's theory of thinking. *Psychoanal. Q.*, 82:323–360.
Davies, J. M. (1998). Multiple perspectives on multiplicity. *Psychoanal. Dialogues*, 8:195–206.
Davies, J. M. & Frawley, M. G. (1994). *Treating the Adult Survivor of Childhood Sexual Abuse: A Psychoanalytic Perspective.* New York, NY: Basic Books.
Dowling, S. (1982). Dreams and dreaming in relation to trauma in childhood. *Int. J. Psychoanal.*, 63:157–166.
Faimberg, H. (2005). *The Telescoping of Generations: Listening to the Narcissistic Links Between Generations.* London: Routledge.
Fonagy, P. (2008). A genuinely developmental theory of sexual enjoyment and its implications for psychoanalytic technique. *J. Amer. Psychoanal. Assn.*, 56:11–36.
Frankiel, R., ed. (1994). *Essential Papers on Object Loss.* New York, NY: New York Univ. Press.
Freud, S. (1900). The Interpretation of Dreams. *S.E.*, 4/5.
——— (1917). Mourning and melancholia. *S.E.*, 14.
Fromm, M. G. (2012). *Lost in Transmission: Studies of Trauma Across Generations.* London: Karnac.
Gottlieb, R. M. (1994). The legend of the European vampire: object loss and corporeal preservation. *Psychoanal. Study Child*, 49:465–480.
Grand, S. (2000). *The Reproduction of Evil: A Clinical and Cultural Perspective.* Hillsdale, NJ: The Analytic Press.
Katz., G. (1998). Where the action is: the enacted dimension of analytic process. *J. Amer. Psychoanal. Assn.*, 46:1129–1167.
——— (2002). Missing in action: the enacted dimension of analytic process in a patient with traumatic object loss. In *Symbolization and Desymbolization: Essays in Honor of Norbert Freedman,* ed. R. Lasky. New York, NY: Other Press, pp. 407–430.
——— (2011). Trauma in action: the enacted dimension of analytic process in a third-generation Holocaust survivor: discussion of "Secretly Attached, Secretly Separate." In *A New Freudian Synthesis: Clinical Process in the Next Generation,* ed. A. B. Druck, C. Ellman, N. Freedman & A. Thaler. London: Karnac, pp. 239–247.
——— (2014). *The Play within the Play: The Enacted Dimension of Psychoanalytic Practice.* London: Routledge.
Kern, J. (1987). Transference neurosis as a waking dream: notes on a clinical enigma. *J. Amer. Psychoanal. Assn.*, 35:337–366.
Laub, D. & Auerhahn, N. C. (1993). Knowing and not knowing massive psychic trauma: forms of traumatic memory. *Int. J. Psychoanal.*, 74:287–302.
Le Fanu, J. S. (1871). *Carmilla,* ed. K. Costello-Sullivan. Syracuse, NY: Syracuse Univ. Press, 2013.
Levenson, E. A. (1972). *The Fallacy of Understanding. An Inquiry into the Changing Structure of Psychoanalysis.* New York, NY: Basic Books.
——— (1983). *The Ambiguity of Change: An Inquiry into the Nature of Psychoanalytic Reality.* New York, NY: Basic Books.
Loewald, H. W. (1960). On the therapeutic action of psycho-analysis. *Int. J. Psychoanal.*, 41:16–33.
——— (1970). Psychoanalytic theory and the psychoanalytic process. *Psychoanal. Study Child*, 25:45–68.
——— (1971). Some considerations on repetition and repetition compulsion. *Int. J. Psychoanal.*, 52:59–66.

——— (1975). Psychoanalysis as an art and the fantasy character of the psychoanalytic situation. *J. Amer. Psychoanal. Assn.*, 23:277–299.

——— (1976). Perspectives on memory. In *Papers on Psychoanalysis*. New Haven, CT: Yale Univ. Press, 1980, pp. 148–173.

Poland, W. S. (1992). Transference: "an original creation." *Psychoanal. Q.*, 61:185–205.

Proust, M. (1981[1913–27]). *Remembrance of Things Past,* trans. C. K. S. Moncrieff, T. Kilmartin & A. Mayor. New York, NY: Random House.

Sandler, J. (1976). Countertransference and role-responsiveness. *Int. Rev. Psychoanal.*, 3:43–47.

Singer, J. A. & Conway, M. A. (2011). Reconsidering therapeutic action: Loewald, cognitive neuroscience, and the integration of memory's duality. *Int. J. Psychoanal.*, 92:1183–1207.

Smith, H. F. (2000). Conflict: see under dissociation. *Psychoanal. Dialogues*, 10:539-550.

Stern, D. B. (2009). *Partners in Thought: Working with Unformulated Experience, Dissociation, and Enactment.* New York, NY: Routledge.

Stoker, B. (2000 [1897]). *Dracula*. Mineola, NY: Dover Publications.

Vivona, J. M. (2003). Embracing figures of speech: the transformative potential of spoken language. *Psychoanal. Psychol.*, 20:52–66.

——— (2006). From developmental metaphor to developmental model: the shrinking role of language in the talking cure. *J. Amer. Psychoanal. Assn.*, 54:877–902.

——— (2009). Embodied language in neuroscience and psychoanalysis. *J. Amer. Psychoanal. Assn.*, 57:1327–1360.

Wilson, N. (2000). A psychoanalytic contribution to psychic vampirism: a case vignette. *Amer. J. Psychoanal.*, 60:177–186.

Yassa, M. & Smith, S. (2000). Vampirism, depression, and symbolization: an analysis of the film *Interview with the Vampire*. *Scandinavian Psychoanal. Rev.*, 23:174–192.

Chapter 5

Do we find or lose ourselves in the negative?[1]

Jade McGleughlin

Abstract

This chapter pools the language of psychoanalysis with other disciplines to illuminate the very real and ephemeral experience of working with patients who experience states of nonbeing. Using the powerful imagery of Francesca Woodman's photographs, my patient and I enter the breach in her mind that trauma creates. Barthes, Benjamin, and art criticism enable me to relate to my patient's condition of trying to exist suspended between life and death.

> Language has unmistakably signified that memory is not an instrument for the exploration of the past, but rather its scene . . . memory must not proceed by way of narrative, much less by way of reports, but must rather assay its spade, epically and rhapsodically in the most rigorous sense, in ever new places and, in the old ones, to delve into ever deeper layers.
>
> Walter Benjamin (Jennings, Eiland and Smith, 1999)

What is coming

Trauma speaks in unknown languages, a confusion of tongues, enigmatic behaviors. What is unsymbolized hides, erupts, displaces, confuses, creating interruptions, leaving gaps. The recognition of certain trauma is marked less by the trauma and its symbolic representation than by a gap trauma creates—what Cathy Caruth (1996) calls "a breach in the mind's experience of time, self, and the world" (p. 4). This breach, often experienced as a state of nonbeing, may be central to certain kinds of early trauma, because "the space of unconsciousness is what paradoxically, preserves the trauma" (p. 62). Unconsciousness or the breach itself, the breach in the mind, is what comes to characterize our subjective experience.

How do we know or register a patient's states of nonbeing, or what I call present absence, and how do we clinically engage the phenomena? Our most familiar impulse is to understand, know, name, and represent trauma in language, but such an impulse to close the gap of traumatic experience may be violating, a terrible erasure and misrecognition of patients who live the breach, whose present absence is a testimony to the gaps in their subjectivity. How do we engage a self-state with little experience of body, time, or history? Is there a linguistic requiem for a psychic gap?

In the work I will present, I had to unlearn my ability to see and name trauma as "something." Instead I entered what I call a negative enactment, which brought the experience of felt absence into reflective consciousness. In the language of Pontalis (1999), I had to "permit the horizon of the object to appear in its immediacy, to allow the invisible to make its appearance through that which is visible" (p. 337). Using the powerful imagery of Francesca Woodman's photographs, an artist who committed suicide at 22 leaving a body of ghostly images, my patient and I were able to find a vehicle to recognize and represent the present absence that haunted her and her treatment and symbolized her being suspended between life and death. Seeing Woodman's photographs in the context of our work together, my patient was able to register and later reflect with me on previously invisible aspects of her experience. I have included several of Woodman's photographs in an effort to participate with Woodman in "inventing an iconography of the invisible/unknowable" (Keller, 2013, p. 177). This chapter is also about a certain kind of listening, which this patient required, not listening *for* the breach but listening *from* the breach in the mind's experience.

In order to bring you into these experiences of a present absence and negative enactment, I have written about our clinical work partially in the "enactive mode" (Naiburg, in press) so that the text "performs or enacts its meaning" (p. ix). For instance I shift my patient's name (you will see naming is a crucial representation of coming into being) in order to evoke her shifting sense of selfhood. I imagined I would use one name to indicate a way she had historically named herself and another to evoke her emerging self-representation but the convention seemed too linear to capture her flux and multiplicity and so I interchange them. I write this way, and also with limited narrative structure and a minimum of scaffolding, not to frustrate you but so that you might experience the mix up of what is unsymbolized and also beginning to be represented. I use a collage of different experiences, atmospheres, registers, and voices, which are necessary for me to convey my process of psychoanalytic witness to trauma. I depart from my familiar relational language and theorists because I am trying to evoke metaphorically (not necessarily theoretically) the idea of something that felt foreign.[2] This paper also implicitly challenges, with Bromberg (1998), the idea of whether closing the gaps is the therapeutic ambition. Instead, I am inviting a kind of being with that might require the calling up and bearing of one's own gaps and ghosts as it did mine.

The case: what is represented

My patient comes to me about ten years ago, does well in the world but feels little agency or subjectivity. I am her second important analyst in 25 years. She tells the story like this. When she is small, her father disappears and a frantic search takes place. While they waited and time stood still, she spun wildly around with her back pressed against a tilt of a world. She says she was sick with vertigo, alone. When he is tracked down months later, he is dead: he has blown his brains out. She is told he died of a heart attack and he is rarely spoken of again. She doesn't remember him and doesn't care. Her mother is all that matters, her only horizon. She's a ship's cook and is gone at sea for long periods of time. She comes back every few weeks and pronounces the world safe and leaves again. My patient cannot catch a breath with her mother's comings and goings. Her mother is a sailor who sailed the seven seas. She is no Helen. And the mud-filled flat she left her to is no Troy. Her mother is a cursing sailor but also the sirens' call. My patient knows that call, lies on that island in that sea, not tied to the mast, not tethered at all. She has no coordinates. She tells me, "I have only empty sacks." She has no home inside. No compass. No guide. The dead are not allowed to speak. They do not anchor an end. They cannot be located (Winterson, 2011).[3]

She tells me this history, because she knows it matters; she's a shrink, but she's not much interested in dredging the past.

The problem of naming/the first sign of the breach

I am disoriented from the beginning. My patient doesn't want me to say her name. If we name her, we will crush her. I learn over time naming demarcates a presence that implies she's been here. If she signs something, like consent, it means she won't be here in the future (Derrida, 1988). It's a dilemma. She's slightly out of all names, slightly out of the frame, like the lipstick of my favorite schizophrenic. I think it's not quite on her lips. Too bright, just slightly fuzzy. An old woman smoking from two mouths at once. But the pink pink colored outside the lines is on right. Tight. That's the funny thing, the rub. Or the stick. That's there too. The fag, the smoke. The pathos, doubled. The doublings of loss. Then and now? The doubleness of death—first her father, then, practically, her mother. It's worse than being crosseyed. It's the face that smears, and smudges. The double.

She's ephemeral, ethereal. Just past my grasp. Every time I think I see her, she's gone. She is, there is, something always moving, sliding away. Now she tells me, ten years later, "Write the paper. Let's see what you can see."

"How do I call you?"

Unexpectedly, she says, "Call me Martin." Martin asks for this name for her disguise.

"Martin? It will be distracting. Gender is not at the center. They will think you are a boy or that the paper is somehow about . . . "

"About trans?"

I say, "Why confuse things?"

She says, "Don't be so literal. Aren't you the analyst? The paper is about trans. About crossings, crossings from the dead. Call me Martin with an (a)."

" Martan? Martina?"

She groans. "Martin with an (a). Write it." But I write Marin. "What about that?"

"You wish," she says. "Marin. Like marine. Like the ocean, like blue, like water. Flow. It's Martin. With an (a). Make no mistake." She wants the (a) outside the name.

Now I write Matin without fail. It takes me a while to see it's French for morning. Matin. Our perpetual nonmourning. Later still, I realize in wanting to call her Matin, I have left out the "r." Without the capability to be. I am. You R. But she's not. That's the point. Or one of them. In the treatment Martin with an (a) was never really there to be named. It's not just about this chapter. As a child, she was called "Nay-Nay." As a noun—a denial or refusal. As a declarative—an emphatic form of NO. Nay-Nay. And in that sing-song childlike first rename, made by a sibling on a subway train (she insists she was named on the subway when her sister turned to see her carriage stuck in the door of the car and began shouting her unpronounceable name, "Nay-Nay"), the beloved nickname and what it signifies sit side by side.

She doesn't ever tell me the name before that name. Naming and constituting **are** the problem. It is taming, pinning down. It locates her as a thing, in the third person, out there in the grid of language. Without a name, Matin conveys her sense of not being. "To be without a name is to be without form or qualities, without shadows, without dreams, without imagination, without a soul" (Himes, 2012, p.16).

Now all these years later there is a firmness with which she wants Martin with an (a). In the context of our relationship, the (a) is something that wasn't there before and alters the negation in ways that remain unclear but must matter (Raniere, 2012, personal communication). This isn't just about what has not been represented but is instead something that hasn't existed. Its nonexistence emerges in hazy ways that are now captured by representing it in terms of symbolization. We are beginning to know some part of Martin that has yet to come into being.

When I write the "a" (she wants the small a, Lacan's object a, the lack, the hole at the center of the symbolic order[4]), I cast it in parenthesis. Unconsciously, I write it as something separate but adjoined. A construction, not quite a conjunctive. The construction is a site of her wanting. In naming herself with me, she is trying to say "I." In saying "I," she is attempting to become a subject of self-reference who is also in relation to others, in relation to me.[5] She is looking for me to be a "you" in relation to whom that "I" could come into being. Then she could secure an "I" in the place of language (Morris, 2013, personal communication).

She is coming in from the periphery of life, making a bridge to an other. She wants a name with me. "It matters what name we choose, we make. People lose their names who lie dead on the field of battle . . . " (Mantel, 2009, p.147). In the beginning of the treatment, I am hopeful we can name her. We will slow down the frame. We will see.

What's in clear (sight)

In my speech on graduating from psychoanalytic training in 2002, I write about Richard Avedon's exhibit at the Metropolitan Museum in New York and the way he captures, in each photograph, something surprising, unfamiliar, not yet seen or known by either the subjects of his pictures or by us, the viewers, even as we contemplate familiar cultural icons (Hambourg and Fineman, 2002). Each portrait is a transformation of someone we thought we knew, redescribed and reconfigured. How did he invent, create, some might say, find, these extraordinary vital parts we know without knowing?

We are told Avedon attends to his sitter with his whole being, watching and sensing viscerally, mirroring and responding to the slightest shifts in his body image, facial expression, and gesture. I thought then portrait making seemed like good relational psychoanalysis. "The portrait is always a solution of the objective and the subjective, the prepared and the improvised, the self and the other"(Hambourg and Fineman, 2002, p.16). Like the psychoanalyst, the portrait maker sees something, catches the element of surprise with his sitter and then, with his vivid portrait, he shows what has been seen. Avedon's portraits seemed to do this.

Something can be seen, new within a single frame.

I am thinking with no shortage of my own omnipotence; I too will reach into the deepest parts of myself, like Avedon, and I will be fully alive and present to the meeting of Matin. I will, like a keen photographer slowing the aperture, capture something surprising, unfamiliar, not yet seen or known. My picture taking will show her her mind with my binocular bi-ocular vision such that we will transform, redescribe, and reconfigure her. We will hold the tension between what is seen and the potential life held by the unconscious. Avedon, with his sure frames and points of departure, with time and space neatly fixed and aligned, with a me and a you, a now and a then, can be bold in black and white. Something else entirely between two people can take shape. But Martin with an (a) does not take shape. Nothing contours. A certain indeterminancy of being—a liminality—something hard to see, to symbolize, exists between us. Something that cannot be seen returns to us again and again, a mobious strip. A no scene. There is no portrait of Matin or Martin or Martin with an (a). Certainly no frame. I can't describe her, fix her, know her. And certainly I cannot show her.

Martin with an (a) is quite sped up really—more like a flipbook. Some images exist, haunt, but it's the pages moving quickly that give you the feel, the story line, the hurrying. A sense of her aura. Her orange aura.

Here is a condensed example from the very beginning of treatment. I cringe to read it. You will note how structured the dialogue is. Open-ended inquiries like "Tell me more" are not useful to Martin. Still, you can see the problem of my trying to "mirror" or "understand." Martin feels pinned like a bug.

In speaking about her mother, Martin with an (a) says, "I wanted to make her life better."

Me: "To be able to make her life better."
Martin: "No. Not able."
I destabilize *her* when I extend by even a word or two, and she bristles.
Martin: "No . . . not able to make it better. I didn't want to be able. It was too much. I felt relief when she remarried. I wasn't totally responsible for her. But then she was gone again with him."
Me: "Relief but gone again and lost to you."
Martin: "No. She was around. She was very involved with me. She was at the center of my life."
Me: "She was at the center. (Long pause.) She meant the world to you."
Martin: "No, not really. Well, we were very close. Her husband was angry I was so much like her."
Me: "Being close meant being like her?"
Martin: (Glares). "No. Jesus." (Long pause—Martin 'goes blank.') Later she says, "It was about going to her. Being with her."
Me: "Being with her."
Martin: "No, not really. He was there." (Dissociation)

Her negation does not feel like resistance though it reads like it. She does not recognize a truth she opposes; she recognizes no truth in what I offer.

She does not, indeed cannot, allow herself to see herself in a state of "alienaction" (Green, 1998, p. 652). The image would be too terrifying. She's not fighting me. She feels internally persecuted, pinned down, and desperate. Each reflection terrifies her—is wrong, partial, enraging, can't be thought about. The effort to know or name through words is not yet possible. I wonder: Has the breach caused a "radical denial of the primordial mind" (p. 652)? My reflection threatens her, as if I had erased something in my seeing and in establishing a thing to be seen. To "see" something definable, or any reflection that attempts to understand her experience, is to NOT understand the erasure within her. Before Martin with an (a) had a name, she cannot bear my "naming" her or her experience. Martin with an (a) wants an analyst who knows how to unname—to be with her both in and outside her experience of a present absence (Morris, 2012, personal communication, drawn from Harold Bloom). She will teach me that naming trauma as a "what," as something that can be represented, is a betrayal. Trauma does not reside in events but in "the breach in the mind's experience" (Caruth, 1996, p. 4). And, it is also true that attunement betrays the profound singularity built into the experience of trauma (Stolorow, 2007).

In a more everyday register, we never quite see ourselves (or each other). The seeing of one's self as a "what" is the problem. I am reminded of those disturbing double takes I experience as I catch a glimpse of the reflection of my face in a store window, and the woman I see isn't me. I experience the same kind of double take interpersonally when I dare to bring my solitary experience to another, and what I see reflected back surprises me or is not the me I recognize. Martin with an (a) felt the same disconnect when the self I mirrored back to her was not the self she knew. When trauma's breach is experienced alone, when the wounding of catastrophe is constituted in isolation, any attempt to move that experience into intersubjective space betrays the experience of having been isolated. Intersubjectivity, then, was not only initially difficult but also, paradoxically, another betrayal (Nguyen, 2012).

We are in a dilemma. Witnessing someone's story or no story can betray the profound singularity built into the experience of trauma. Yet, without an other to reconstitute an experience of selfhood, the rupture in human connection that is often at the core of profound trauma cannot be repaired. It's captured in our naming quandary. Being constituted in the mind of the other is a tyranny for Martin, yet naming holds the potential for her to constitute herself with me. We live in this paradox.

Martin longs to be constituted as Martin with an (a), but the name remains not quite complete, the (a) hanging off. She has no fixed identity or sense of subjectivity a name would imply. For now she resists the power of the gaze to implicate a "her" that is not yet subjectively there. She wants to keep her aura. What then is the aura? "A strange tissue of space and time: the unique apparition of a distance, however near it may be" (Benjamin, 2008, p. 23). This aura suggests liminality of time and space that can't be reduced. She would think, like Barthes tells us in *Camera Lucida* (1980), in the very representation of the image itself, when the picture is taken, there is a death, including the death of the aura. If I see her, it will feel like a kind of murder—"the stripping of a veil from the object, the destruction of the aura" (Benjamin, 2008, p. 23). Representing feels like robbing or worse, death.

Treatment history

The treatment is rocky. First there is curiosity, then devaluing, contempt, scorn. A few years later a love develops, a hunger, but the longing is terrifying, and Matin slips away into deep retreat. The tumults of those years focus on her mother, on the emergence of that chaotic relationship into ours. Connecting moments are followed by her contempt, fear. My words often fail to reach her. The transference is positive, disrupted, negative. The treatment is rich, sometimes disastrous. But we survive, and in surviving all this, something else comes into being, delicate and ordinary. It's hard to recognize it as psychoanalysis, but I think we are laying down track, rigging the boat. Maybe some might call this transitional space or a facilitating environment. The capacity for relating as two subjects is rare. Matin is not separate. There are few interpretations, not much reflective analytic process but a slow kind of simple daily life lived in the analytic frame. There is acknowledgment, witness, and shared rhythm. If we lived it in the world, we would be slowly walking side-by-side or cooking or maybe looking out together from a bench towards a sea. (For the missing mother?) Perhaps we each know "the subtleness of the sea; how its most dreaded creatures glide under water, unapparent for the most part, and treacherously hidden beneath the loveliest tints of azure" (Melville, 1851, p. 301), but we talk of "Where to store fur and how to treat hair" (St. Vincent Millay, 1917, p. 41). I am containing, holding inside, those monsters under the sea. I am thinking of Milner's concept extended from Winnicott's ideas of unintegration in which an environment must be reliably safe to allow the subject to flounder in "absence-mindedness" (Farhi, 2010, p. 488). I am holding inside of me the image of Martin with an (a) beginning to BE.

The image: What we do see

"A person, scattered in space and time, is no longer a woman but a series of events in which we can throw no light, a series of insoluble problems."[6]

How do we represent what cannot be represented? In the seventh year of the treatment, I go to the Guggenheim Museum to see Francesca Woodman's solo show. Woodman (1958–1981) has become one of the most studied and influential photographers of the late twentieth century. She began photographing at 13 and committed suicide by jumping from a building when she was 22. Many of her photographs have Woodman "haunting the boundaries, edging out of or coming into the frame, almost slipping through the surface of representation, away from us, toward us, coming out of the back of the picture, blending into the walls like a maladroit tyro ghost" (Townsend, 2006, p. 7).

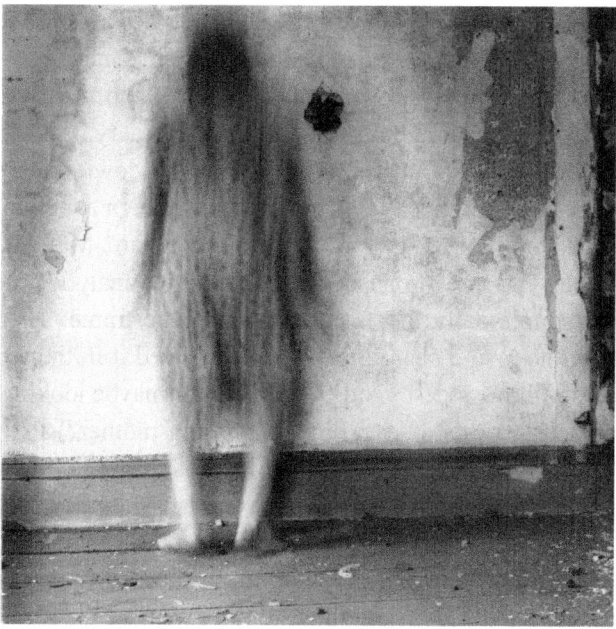

Figure 5.1 Polka Dots, Providence, Rhode Island. Courtesy of George and Betty Woodman.

Despite her perpetual presence in the photographs as model, "Woodman is always on the verge of disappearance. Her face is most often obscured from the camera: on the rare occasion when she fixes us squarely in her gaze, the effect is riveting but disquietly unrevealing (Keller, 2013, p. 178). "Not only is she both subject and author in her works (as both the analyst and patient are), but also she intentionally alludes to the representation of self within pictures . . . while simultaneously suggesting a disjunction between the self and its identity, and between the body and the self" (p. 178). I sense Martin with an (a), like Woodman's tyro ghosts, is also gliding, slipping into things, other self-states, other graves.

Critics write that Woodman's work challenges the certainties of photography: "The fixing of time and space that might otherwise be understood as its most fundamental characteristic" (Townsend, 2006, p. 7). She does this ironically through the use of a medium that is meant to represent what is most indisputably there (Townsend, 2006). Yet Woodman's art is "preoccupied with showing us that what is most indisputably there is uncertain, not fixed in time, filled with hesitation and the displacement of forms . . . she is evading the fixity that technical limits of photography would impose" (Townsend, 2006, p. 7). In challenging the permeability of boundaries in actual space and time in visual representation, Woodman draws our attention to the liminality of personhood (Keller, 2013, p. 177).

It is what Martin does too.

Martin, like Woodman, seems to exude "a profound ambivalence—a simultaneous refusal and yearning to be constituted in the field of vision as an object of desire" (Sundell, 2003, p. 53). For Martin with an (a), and for Woodman, being looked at and being seen emerge as boundary disturbances (Raymond, 2010). Woodman conveys this through her use of physical space. She is always moving our gaze, tilting the frame, obscuring, blurring the image, slowing the negative. Slowing down the aperture. Martin does it by shape shifting, moving away. Each time I think we have come to shared meaning, I am wrong. If Woodman uses a medium that is meant to represent what is most indisputably there to show what is not there, Martin too creates this disjuncture in our experience of her by shifting self-states, disappearing from where she is just minutes earlier, erasing her mind, thinking of nothing, becoming blank.

One critic suggests Woodman's images are her own fort/da game[7]—an attempt to master her own state of nonbeing (my word): The casting out

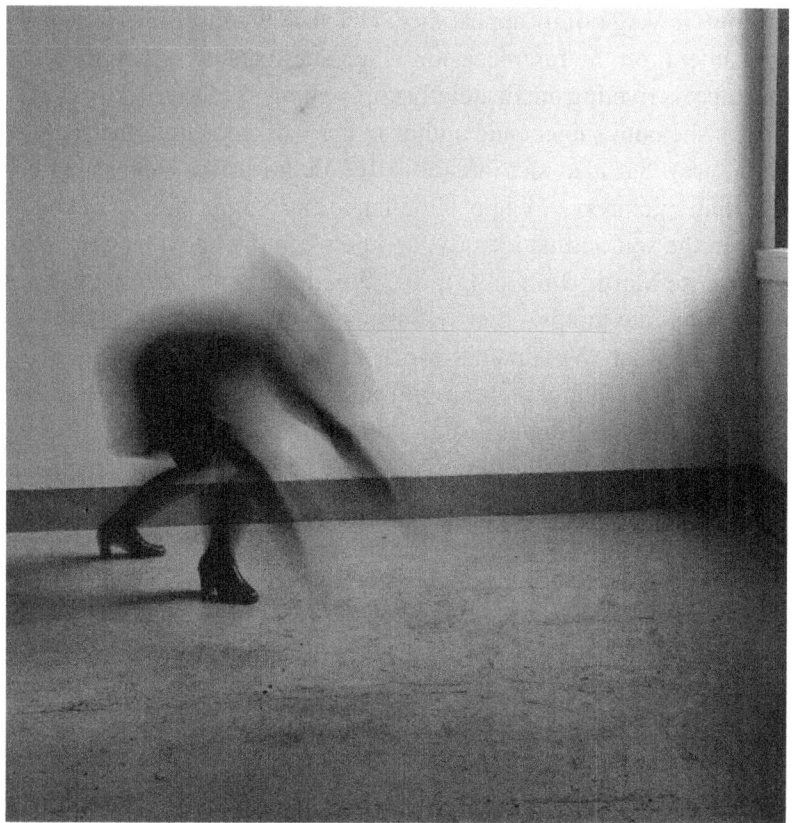

Figure 5.2 Space, [2] Providence, Rhode Island 1976. Courtesy of George and Betty Woodman.

and reeling in of images that both grasp self-image and offer access to an image of her own imagelessness (Phelan, 2002).

Martin with an (a) plays fort/da too. For both women, psychoanalysis and photographic self-portraiture respectively could "promise <u>knowledge</u> of the self, [but] there is a resistant enigma of vision, a non-entity describing itself as an entity" (Phelan, 2002, p. 987). Woodman's critics note, "In their paradoxical blurring and emphasizing of the body, Woodman's pictures pose questions about the limits of subjectivity in materiality" (Raymond, 2010, p. 2). The aura of Martin with an (a) and the images in Woodman's self-portraits "obliterate our capacities as viewers to identify with them as subject(s)" (p. 987).

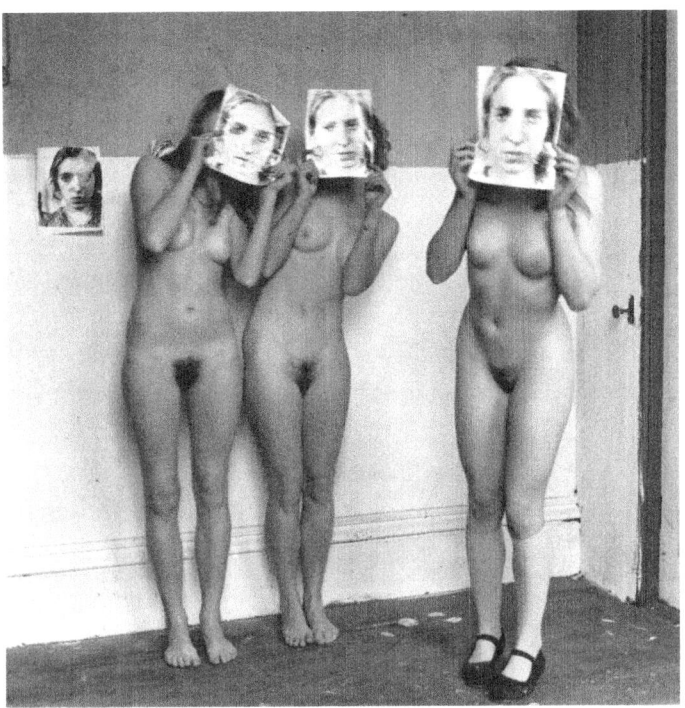

Figure 5.3 About Being My Model, Providence 1976. Courtesy of George and Betty Woodman.

Potentially like Freud's grandson, who is attempting to master his mother's comings and goings and hold a presymbolic image of presence in her absence, Woodman and Martin's appearing and disappearing are potentially attempting to represent and hold something that is just beginning to be developed and known - a sense of internal absence in presence. I am taken with the way both women seem to be drawing our attention to a kind of liminal presence that can look like fragmentation but might be pointing us towards something else. Martin, in her appearances and disappearances, seems to be developing a way to represent what is an emergent sense of what's alien within her.

Woodman herself calls some of her blurred motion figures "ghost pictures," and Raymond (2010) notes one of her early curators, Ferris (2003), chose to exhibit her photos alongside the spirit photographs made in the nineteenth and early twentieth centuries, in which the glass

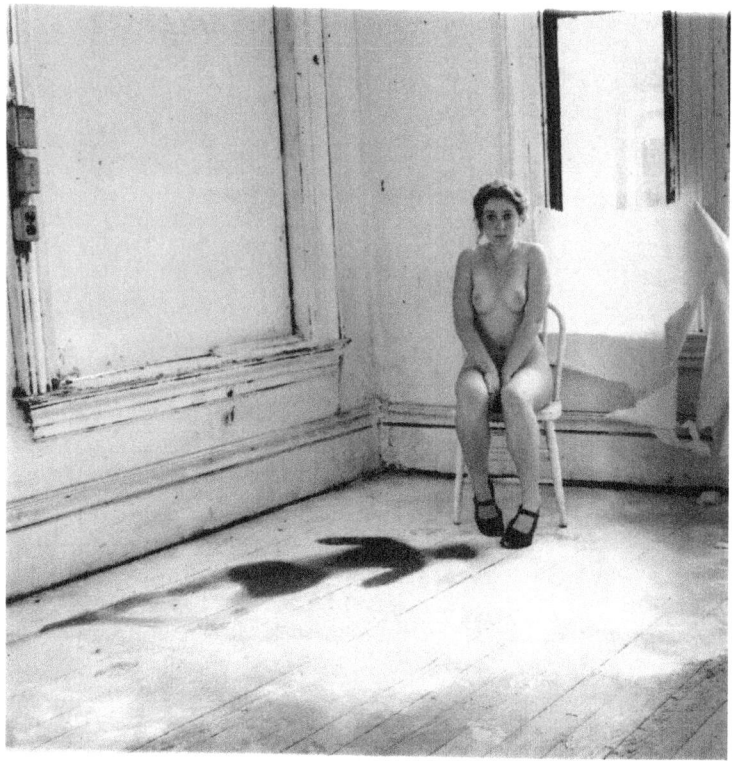

Figure 5.4 Untitled, Providence 1976. Courtesy of George and Betty Woodman.

plates were altered and double exposures were used to trick mourners into believing the image of the departing soul had been captured as proof of life after death. If Woodman is trying to photograph something that doesn't exist, as Krauss (1986) suggests, is Martin trying to signal the ways in which she doesn't exist and or is she trying to allude to the ways she is potentially filled up, forced to live out the "devastating half life" of her dead (Abraham and Torok, 1984, p. 167)? I had been thinking about Martin with an (a)'s shifting self-states or states of nonbeing as about her difficulty inhabiting herself. Now I begin to wonder if a second phenomenon is with us, the possibility that the ghosts of her father inhabit her. Does the (a) that hangs off Martin's name represent her missing self-states or could it also be Martin's ghost or phantom or father? All this plays in my mind.

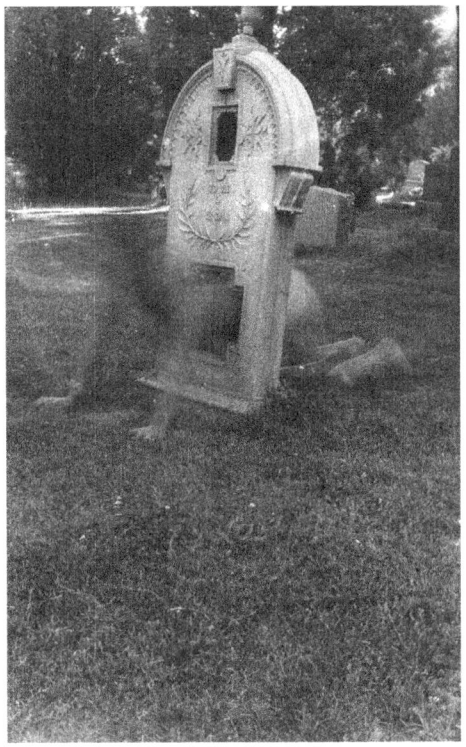

Figure 5.5 Untitled, Boulder Colorado 1972–1975. Courtesy of George and Betty Woodman.

Certainly Woodman's photographs seem to challenge the idea of "photographs as documents of the past that bear witness . . . and substantiate the existence of experiences" (Blessing and Tottman, 2011, p. 11). Instead they are spectral images that might, as Barthes (1980) suggests, create a rehearsal for death, allowing the viewer access to the ongoing psychic work of mourning. But for me they also evoke the loss of never having come fully into being—of being neither dead nor alive. It might be as critic Keller (2013) notes that Woodman is ultimately commanding the photograph not to destabilize identity but rather, for its sheer usefulness as a tool, to reveal identity's fractionary quality. But I think there is more. Woodman inhabits another space. She herself writes that the task of her photographs (Phelan, 2002) was to allow her to locate "where I fit in this odd geometry of time."[8] Hmm.

The Showing

Perhaps in unconscious association to the work that is between us (in the field), I mention I have been to the Woodman show in New York. Martin decides to go see the show, travels there, and has a powerful experience. She begins to photograph Woodman's photographs. In the following weeks Martin and I look at those photographs and some books of Woodman's work. She brings me other photographs from the web. In session, we speak about what we see separately and together in the photographs. We wonder why are Woodman's pictures so liminal? Why is she ethereal, floating, ungrounded? What was Woodman trying to see, what space was she trying to inhabit? Did Woodman have ghosts that haunted her? What happened before she jumped from the building? What is the meaning of the ways she plays with the boundaries between life and death?

We don't know if Woodman imagined her death, staged it, or wanted us to see, in Barthes (1980) words, a rehearsal for it. We don't know if her photographs speak to us from the grave as Barthes implies is possible. But I do believe Woodman has planted what LaPlanche and Pontalis (1967) call an enigmatic message (unconsciously as all enigmatic messages are implanted) for each of us who wears her closely to decipher with our own afterwardness, our own now-conferred understanding of what was happening before she suicided and now that we know her death.[9] Something stirs in our unconscious. Martin says she likes the indeterminancy of the photos, the way Woodman is never static and also always somewhere else. She tells me she objects to the world of reproductions, where the ephemeral is lost. It's why she doesn't like interpretations. She doesn't want to be anybody's picture, anybody's copy. In these photos she sees something that interests her. Woodman's aura and her own. Martin's camera trained on Woodman's camera allows another vision.

> Clearly, it is another nature, which speaks to the camera as compared to the eye. 'Other' above all in the sense that a space informed by human consciousness gives way to a space informed by the unconscious . . . It is through the camera that we first discover the optical unconscious, just as we discover the instinctual unconscious through psychoanalysis.
> (Benjamin, 2008, p.37)

What Woodman creates and Martin (a) and I see through the optical unconscious is a kind of ghost-like figure who cannot be stabilized, rooted, pinned down. Is Woodman a phantom? Is Martin? Am I? We don't know yet who we see, who we feel, what we know. We feel how haunted Woodman was and we feel her haunting us.

As Benjamin (2008) notes:

> Photography can bring out aspects of the original that are accessible only to the lens (which is adjustable and can easily change viewpoint) but not to the human eye ... With the close up, space expands. With slow motion, movement is extended and just as enlargement not merely clarifies what we see, ... but brings to light entirely new structures of matter, slow motion not only reveals familiar aspects of movements but discloses quite unknown aspects within them—aspects which do not appear as the retarding of natural movements, but has a curious gliding, floating character of their own.
>
> (p. 37)

Woodman has captured unknown aspects of Martin—what lies outside the normal spectrum of sense impressions. Like a gift from a psychotic, ghost, or angel, Woodman offers us another kind of real—the space between presence and absence. She has made the invisible visible and the shapeless, a form. When Martin sees Woodman's gliding, disappearing, fragmenting, negative self, we come to know she sees something new.

The Enactment

The more I read about Woodman, the more surprised I become. The body of criticism on Woodman's work is curiously antipsychoanalytic. Biographical details are concrete, insubstantial, and provided as though without psychic relevance. Even the more psychoanalytic critics demonstrate a significant disavowal of the meaning of her suicide. In fact, in almost everything I've read, no reference to her suicide is made or else it is seriously underplayed. The critics reject interpretations of her work as biographical revelation—troubled psyche, youthful suicide—and instead focus on her genius, her aesthetics, "the question of whether aesthetic effects are tricks, illusions, or eruptive markers of the real" (Raymond, 2010, p. 2). In the first catalogues and critical reviews of her work, a conscious decision was made not to mention her death (Phelan, 2002, p. 984). Almost all of the critics plead for us not to interpret her art through her suicide or reduce art to autobiography or symptom. I understand. Still, I am surprised, as if repetitive, insistent images and themes of liminality have little meaning, and psyche has no place. Each critic consciously refuses the idea that a person who commits suicide is necessarily in some anguish that has relevance to her work. In the only piece about the meaning of death in Woodman's art, Phelan, a critic I greatly admire and who is critical of the denial of the meaning of Woodman's death for her art, indicates that her suicide did not necessarily signal a tragedy but a kind of tentative achievement, even her gift to us by helping us imagine a future in which she is no longer there (Phelan, 2002, p. 984)! With this exception, the more I read about Woodman, the more it seemed as if the effort to understand Woodman's death is obscured from the viewer. The critics seem to be trying to erase the difference between life and death as if they are saying her death was immaterial to her art.

When I tell this story to a colleague, he notes my big affect, my outrage. He pushes me to think about why I am so disturbed. I cannot join the critics in this apparent disavowal of death.

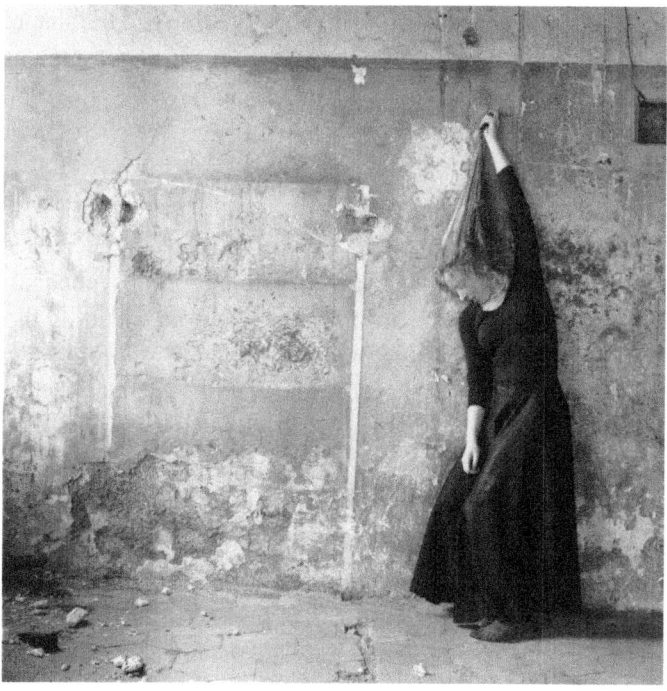

Figure 5.6 Untitled, Rome 1977–1978. Courtesy of George and Betty Woodman.

If we think of these contrasting views, mine and the critics', as a visual scene, it is what Barthes (1980) calls the punctum,[10] the thing that starts internal agitation, the detail that stands out, that punctures and pierces, that helps us see (Morris, 2012, personal communication). Suddenly, the meaning of erasing the boundary between life and death registers inside of me like a shock that disturbed my dissociation of my own ghosts, of my liminality. While the disavowal, denial, or repression that Martin and I shared about the death of our fathers was relevant, it was not what was calling to us most. Metaphorically it was her own and maybe my difficulty inhabiting life. This punctum stunned me into seeing what had not been in my sight. Disturbed and awakened, I could begin to formulate from the site of my traumatic history both my liminality and Martin's. I had not been able to see how Martin hovered between life and death. The enactment with the Woodman art critics catapulted me into reflection about my own grip of a sensory experience of present absence.

Knowing the difference between life and death

This moment in the treatment marks a turning point in the work, where I begin to sense my disavowal of not knowing the difference between life and death. It is indeed my moving away from known losses, Martin's and my own, into my own liminal state that shifted what each of us could know. We leave the realm of "understanding," and each enter the site of our unknown individual trauma, learning to forgo identification with the other to be with ourselves *and* each other in our "emphatic unsettlement" (LaCapra, 2001). We are in a mode of seeing "suggesting one might not know that one is dreaming, or that one might see only without knowing it" (Caruth, 1996, p. 39).

What does this actually look like in the lived experience of the treatment?

It is very hard to say. I am not trying to place the experience beyond phenomenological description, but this kind of other-worldly transmission I speak of does not happen in language or event but punctum. The presence of Woodman's work hangs in the consulting room like ether. It permeates our space in waves, (never locatable) not quite mirage or image but atmosphere. Our much earlier version of "absence-mindedness" (Farhi, 2010, p. 488) in which Martin and I were looking together from a bench towards the sea has given way to something more gripping: We are now in that sea. Whatever was under water, out of sight is with us now as a palpable presence of absence, heavy and disruptive. The sessions are languid, drifty—hard to bear. Sometimes it means both of us, me behind the couch, her on the couch, are joined in a state of floating, somnolent, amorphous experience. I think of somatic reverie and drowning. I don't want to call it unconscious communication exactly, because I think we are creating something new that could not come into being until there was an intersubjective system to house the experience (Stolorow, et al., 1987). We are embodying or enacting the absent past that couldn't be remembered or represented, because it was in excess of our frames of reference (Felman and Laub, 1992). This is what I am calling a negative enactment: that which brings forward an invisible state of unformulated trauma like the negative of the photograph. When "we lose ourselves in the negative" (Pontalis, 1999, p. 898), something opens. As Caruth (1996) notes, the transmission of the unrepresentable happens when the listener is brought into the trauma making us, in Dori Laub's language, "participants and co-owners of the traumatic event" (Leys, 2000, p. 269).

Martin and I begin to know that where ever else she lives, she also lives in the shimmer, in the in-between, in the gap. This is as close to home as any state she knows. And I am a knowing guest.

If there is any concrete change, it's this: Over the next months as Martin and I hold Woodman's images between us, reverie about my dead father surfaces, and I think of my own failure to mark his death and the way that keeps me from fully inhabiting my subjectivity. Simultaneously, references to Martin's father emerge here and there in a dream or association. She might talk of missing, and I might say something like, "Your father went missing and has always been missing," and Martin acknowledges the psychic relevance. Or she dreams of herself lying on parchment paper, and if she shifts her weight, the paper will give way to a moving grave, carried on a conveyor belt below her suspended body. What had previously been invisible, and unimaginable, increasingly emerges into images, feelings, and words. In the consulting room time reasserts itself. There becomes a before and an after, a now and a then.

Soon her body, always foreign to her, will also emerge.

We talk. We come to live together the way her trauma was experienced too early to be fully known. We "feel" into what was cliché; that for my patient to lay claim to her own survival, she would have to lay her father to rest (Caruth, 1996). She knows an unbridgeable gap where the missing father went missing and then was missing forever. In this story, missing the moment of his death, she is also unable to recognize the continuation of her life.[11] One strand of my patient's difficulty inhabiting herself and experiencing subjectivity—fundamentally knowing she is alive—may involve her own inability to mark her father's passage from life to death. There was no body, no funeral, no grave, and no acknowledgement that her father was dead. There was no "then" or "after" that marked his death. If her father is not really dead, he cannot be mourned. But to claim life by grasping his death would be to remember him as a living being and lose him again (Caruth, 1995). We wonder: has my patient made her father the part of her that escaped her (Pontalis, 1999)? The small (a)? Rather than experience identification with the dead father, in this frame my patient is possessed by this foreign body that "acquires from within a relentless power, the power of a drive. Words would break the continuity of that line—a total and final separation" (p. 899). Representing the death in words kills the ghost and loses the object. My patient has a dilemma.

My patient's act of survival is "the repeated confrontation with the necessity and impossibility of grasping the threat to her life" (Caruth, 1996, p. 8), the threat that she has not known or has been rigidly disavowed. "Survival becomes, paradoxically, an endless testimony to the impossibility of living" (Caruth, 1996, p. 8). Where memory might be, breach is.

The body brings terror

These shared understandings give way to terror. Ghosts erase the difference between life and death. Now Martin with an (a) begins to feel how her disavowal of her father's suicide has impeded her ability to inhabit herself and how he has simultaneously possessed her. Martin has existed in a kind of melancholic dysthymic wandering in which no one cried out (Caruth, 1996): no body was felt. Disembodied, there was no pain or pleasure. Now her body and the excruciating pain of the trauma she had not consciously experienced return together. There is an awakening. It starts with her breasts. Martin with an (a) tells me she feels her breasts for the first time. She can feel them as erotic objects. As soft shapes beneath her fingers. She never was a breast man. Now with the existence of a body, so do I become alive. She moves towards me.

She writes,

> I wake up in the winter
> I am wearing you tight
> Across my chest where I have felt

> Strange tingling for days and weeks now
> And I mind just a little these pricks of soma rubbing
> Into mind breasts chapped and almost straining across the room to you.

The psychic cache of having breasts is unimaginable. With the breasts, the huge hole of their absence asserts itself. Now anxiety, symptoms, desire, longing. No one said breasts were just for fun. A direct relational element emerges. Can she use me? Am I real? Can she feel me? Will I stay? She thinks not. The return to bodily memory awakens relationality—and trauma.

At the site of Woodman's work, in our eighth year of treatment, Martin's drift gives way to terror. Suddenly Martin is shouting, trembling, sobbing. Martin with an (a)'s father's suicide begins to register through a terrible fear of the future. She begins to feel the terror she must have felt as a small girl as her world collapsed—feelings she could not know then. Each morning she awakens to the certain feeling that everyone she loves will disappear. Psychic reality trumps husband, children, me. We truly are abandoning her. She tells me I won't show up, won't come back, will evaporate. It's painful to separate, to know I will die. She wants promises. Assurances. To be part of my funeral or illness or any other departure she can imagine. She will not be on the outside of death again. She does not know if she can survive the future. The fear of it undoes her. It's the dread of that dismal. It's not a loss she fears. It's a disaster. A whole world shattering. The catastrophe is back as if for the first time—and only now in this strange place and time does it constitute itself. Martin with an (a) had not known the violence of her losses, and their return makes her sweat and shake. It is the traumatic awakening from death into life that is now upon her. My body/mind too feels dread. I hope it is the dread preceding surrender (Ghent, 1990).

Discussion

What really allowed change? Working in the visual register allowed us to know about a state of nonbeing that did not exist in language and originally could not be represented in words. Without being fully conscious of what I was doing, I offered Martin a visual interpretation of her own (metaphoric) liminality. I see now this was an act of figurability in which the analyst "initiates and catalyzes processes that strengthen and or integrate [the patient's] ability to think by strengthening and integrating weakly inscribed psychic elements or giving form to something that was previously unrepresented"

(Levine and Reed, 2012 p. 49). When I bring Woodman's images into the field, I am offering an unthought interpretation in the visual form, and new meaning is generated. I say an unthought interpretation because I was not fully conscious of what I was introducing. Perhaps the images, ideas, and affects existed in a form that was pre-representable. When she and I see them together, something inchoate begins to form and be represented.

I want to notice at least two registers in which change happened. When Martin sees that I have seen a version of her experience of present absence in Woodman's images of liminality, this allows Martin to accept outside sight and see her reflection through my seeing her. My reflection is uncertain, partial, and tentative, and the images themselves suggest something inchoate, blurred, and lurking that feels reflective. These reflections give rise to Martin's unarticulated feelings about her own sense of nonbeing and "makes mental space, emotional states, and their symbolization more possible" (Bonowitz, 2007, p. 631). Martin then uses Woodman as a mirror to constitute an image of herself paradoxically as both a being and a nonbeing, so her "I" can see a version of her "me" (Seligman, 2007, Ogden, 2001). We have created a space between Martin as subject and her experience of herself as someone who can be represented. And when we do, Martin is able to experience her body, and the terror that accompanies the experience of being alive.

But what allows this use of me? Martin can do this, because she thinks that for me to see her as ghost or liminal being, I must have my own ghost(s). This moves us into shared experience, which is necessary for witnessing trauma but not enough in itself. We have moved from object relating to transitional relating (Winnicott, 1969). Martin has, without impingement, discovered her own motility. She reaches, creates, finds a "me" and a "you." Now something more like object use develops. Our relationship is real, vitalized, filled with love and hate.

If we believe trauma was experienced too early in Martin's life and too shockingly/violently to be fully known by her, Martin needs an other with whom to constitute her traumatic history. I am interested anew in Freud's early trauma theory, as reviewed in Caruth (1996), not as theory but as metaphor. He tells us that what is truly striking about the train accident or trauma victim's experience of the event is not so much the forgetting that occurs afterward but rather that the crash victim is never fully conscious during the accident. Caruth emphasizes the temporal aspect of trauma, noting that the fright is not known, because it registers a moment too late when a breach has already occurred. Said another way, traumatic experience is not mediated through a mind and what it represses, because the mind has missed the event. This theory has holes (so to speak). In my view of trauma, moments of disavowal and acknowledgment oscillate; everything is registered, return is never literal, just (Morris, 2012, personal communication[12]). Afterwardness confers meaning. Trauma lands and surfaces from the complexity of all we are and are becoming. Yet as metaphor, something calls to us in this outdated theory. The metaphor of nonbeing may be central to certain kinds of early trauma, because the trauma is experienced only belatedly and indirectly. Because the patient does not own or possess the knowledge of the trauma, and our own truths continually escape us (Felman and Laub, 1992), it is only in the engagement with an other that that trauma becomes constituted. As Caruth (2006) notes, it is the fundamental incomprehensibility at the heart of trauma that necessitates intersubjective entanglement. Without fully grasping the other's or even our own trauma, Martin and I needed each other for each of us to create an opening to establish history and memory. "This speaking and listening, from the site of trauma does not rely . . . on what we simply know of each other, but on what we don't know of our own traumatic pasts" (1996, p. 56). I believe that it is our being in our **own** liminality rather than identifying liminality as a phenomenon we share that allows the intersubjective entanglement to give rise to the creation of memory and representation.

I take away several ideas from this work (some well worn) that startled me in a new way: That seeing trauma as a "what" can easily be experienced as a betrayal; that trauma's breach of the mind alters time and hence one's experience of having a coherent personal history; that while the belatedness of trauma requires an other to constitute a history, paradoxically recognizing difference in addition to bridging otherness through empathy is crucial; and that one needs to speak to the traumatized person from within the site of one's own trauma, from our own inner breach and "unsettled knowledge" rather than from an identification based on the recognition that each has experienced trauma.

Being together not coming together[13]

I want to emphasize this last point. When I am listening to Martin from my own corresponding history of loss, I potentially appropriate her story. I have been alive to the familiar issues of loss and disavowal regarding the death of my own father, but not alive to the way that disavowal left me, metaphorically in my own liminality. I colluded with Martin in not seeing the way she has not been alive, because I was blind to an aspect of my own corresponding liminality.

By using our own known experience as a way to know the other, we may fail to create the necessary interruption in our patient's and our own looping self-narratives. We may need an interruption that surprises— something that is almost like a slap or shock that invites some element of distinction, separateness, and bodily awareness where absence and dissociation have been (Caruth, 1996). The Woodman critics created this dissonance or shock for me and for Martin (a) by their disavowing the significance of her suicide, denying the difference between life and death.

I continue to believe as I wrote in an earlier paper (McGleughlin, 2011) in accord with Slavin (2011) and Lombardi (2005) that when we are willing to travel back to the place of corresponding deficit within ourselves, to struggle with our own internal splits in our effort to reach the other, a channel toward change and transformation may open. I still believe alongside Harris (2009) and others that impasse may loosen when the analyst has access to unbearable affects and is able to metabolize, shift, grieve, change, and speak from this slightly altered state. Still something more was highlighted in this work with Martin with an (a) that I have grasped in a new way. Then I wrote that we had to help our patients in those places we can't yet help ourselves, which I now understand to be our own places of potential. But perhaps it is equally true that our own absences need to be recognized and somehow represented. Martin with an (a) made a demand: to listen not from what I know about my own losses but from the place they have infected me and made me blank. It is in that way when the "referential function of words begins to break down . . . what is transmitted is 'not the normalizing knowledge of the horror but the horror itself'" (Michaels, 1996, p. 8).

Summary

Avedon showed us what we did not know in someone familiar. Woodman helped us recognize our need to see what is not yet there. Morris notes that acknowledging death depends on a willingness to be disturbed. Ultimately, it means being able to distinguish between life and death. Caruth (1996) emphasized the way in which one's own trauma is tied up with the trauma of another and that in the "very possibility and surprise of listening to another's wound," one is able to "bear witness" (p. 3) by creating a platform from which to enter the incomprehensible.

Martin with an (a) and I are still in process. Movement is not linear, more in and out. But we are in the grit of human relating. Yesterday she asks, in the language of Leanh Nguyen (2012), if I know real intimate contact with another mind/body who I have allowed to see me, smell me, know me in my abject fear and pathetic bodily functions?[14] I nod. When I can feel your breathe on my face, my terror smells ripe.

Notes

1 Pontalis, J. B. (1999). Special thanks for their help to Adrienne Harris, Humphrey Morris, David Raniere, Stephen Seligman, and Mal Slavin.
2 There is an extensive dialogue about unformulated experience most prominently explored by Stolorow, Brandchaft, and Atwood's (1987) "prereflective unconscious," Bollas's (1987) "unthought known," Stern's (1983, 1985, 1989) unformulated experience and D. N. Sterns, et al.'s "implicit relational knowing."
3 Winterson cites Romanian scholar Mircea Eliade's ontological as well as geographical notion of home. "Home," he tells us, "is the intersection of two lines—the vertical and the horizontal. The vertical plane has heaven, or the upper world, at one end, and the world of the dead at the other end. The horizontal plane is the traffic of this world, moving to and fro—our own traffic and that of teeming others." Winterson tell us, "Home was a place of order, a place where the order of things comes together—the living and the dead—the spirits of the ancestors and the present inhabitants, and the gathering up and stilling of all the to and fro . . . At worst, a displaced person literally does not know which way is up, because there is no true north. No compass point . . . For the refugee, for the homeless, this lack of crucial coordinate in the placing of the self has severe consequences" (p. 58).
4 Zizek as quoted in Himes, 2012.
5 Saying "I" is occupying – temporarily – the position of the speaker in relation to the "you" who is my addressee. Through the act of nomination, we attempt to become a subject of reference FOR others. Whereas in saying "I," we attempt to become a subject of self-reference, IN RELATION TO others. See Paul Ricouer's, *Oneself As An Other,* which gives an extensive discussion of this distinction. (Morris, 2013, personal communication).
6 Proust, 1923, as quoted in Townsend, 2006, p. 7.
7 Freud writes about his grandson, who in an effort to master his mother's disappearance and return, creates a game where he casts a spool out and reels it backs in, a process critical to the development of continuity in absence. Freud calls this the fort/da game, and it was first discussed in *Beyond The Pleasure Principle*.
8 The phrase appears in Woodman's text written below two photographs in *Some Disordered Interior Geometries*, reproduced in Chris Townsend, *Francesca Woodman* Oxford: Phaidon Press, 2006, p. 238.
9 Unlike Barthes (1980), who finds relief in his dead mother's photograph because it signals that she existed in a time before he was alive, and hence creates the possibility that he can go on after her death, I find no mourning possibilities in these images. Woodman's indeterminacy, her refusal/inability/disinterest in capturing her own still life, her own portrait, a firmly rooted image of herself as alive or dead suggests something must precede our mourning.

10 Elsewhere I have described Barthes' concepts (1980) of studium and punctum in discussing a certain group of well-composed photographs. Perhaps the critics view Woodman's work through the lens of what he calls studium; a visual concept, a way of seeing the image that evokes commitment or interest without acuity; unconcerned desire on the order of liking, not loving; an interest that comes from one's training or culture; a kind of education that allows one to discover the picture taker, the intentions that motivate or animate his practice, but as spectator. I want Woodman's critics to exist, not as spectators on the outside, but as participants. Barthes (1980) is writing about seeing and being seen prior to, or outside of language: studium and punctum are ways of looking and being looked at. They hold the tension between language and image, and indeed there is something in this tension that holds more than speech – that invokes mood and feeling and change.
11 These are ideas formulated from Caruth's reading of the film "Hiroshima Mon Amour" (1961) in *Unclaimed Experience* (2006).
12 See Leys (2000) critique of Caruth's reconceptualization of Freud.
13 Caruth, 1996.
14 Nguyen, (2012) Psychoanalytic Activism.

This chapter first appeared as 'Do We Find or Lose Ourselves in the Negative?' in *Psychoanalytic Dialogues* 25 (2): 214-236, April 2015. Reprinted by permission of Taylor & Francis, LLC and The International Association for Relational Psychoanalysis and Psychotherapy (http://www.iarrp.net).

Bibliography

Abelin, G. (1993). Perdue De Vue: By J.-B. Pontalis. Paris: Gallimard, 1988, 307 pp., Fr 115. *Journal of the American Psychiatric Association*, 41, 897–899.
Abraham, N. and Torok, M. (1994). *The Shell and the Kernel, Volume I*. Chicago, IL and London, England: The University of Chicago Press.
Baker, G., Daly, A., Davenport, N., Larson, L., and Sundell, M. (2003, Summer). Francesca Woodman Reconsidered: A Conversation with George Baker, Ann Daly, Nancy Davenport, Laura Larson and Margaret Sundell. *Art Journal*, 62, 2, 52–67.
Barthes, R. (1980). *Camera Lucida: Reflections on Photography*. New York, NY: Hill and Wang, a Division of Farrar, Straus, and Giroux.
Benjamin, W. (2006). *Berlin Childhood around 1900*. Cambridge, MA and London, England: The Belknap Press of Harvard University Press.
Benjamin, W. (2008). *The Work of Art in the Age of Its Technological Reproducibility and Other Writings on Media*. Cambridge, MA and London, England: The Belknap Press of Harvard University Press.
Blessing, J., Phelan, P., and Trotman, N. (2010). *Haunted: Contemporary Photography, Video, Performance*. New York, NY: Guggenheim Museum.
Bollas, C. (1987). *The Shadow of the Object: Psychoanalysis of the Unthought Known*. New York, NY: Columbia University Press.
Bonowitz, C. (2010). The Interpersonalization of Fantasy: The Linking and De-linking of Fantasy and Reality. *Psychoanalytic Dialogues*, 20, 627–641.
Bromberg, P. (1998). *Standing In The Spaces: Essays on Clinical Process, Trauma and Dissociation*. Hillsdale, NJ: The Analytic Press.
Caruth, C. (1995). *Trauma: Explorations in Memory*. Baltimore, MD: The Johns Hopkins University Press.

Caruth, C. (1996). *Unclaimed Experience: Trauma, Narrative, and History*. Baltimore, MD and London, England: The Johns Hopkins University Press.
Derrida, J. (1988). Signature Event Context. In *Limited Inc*. Evanston, IL: Northwestern University Press.
Farhi, N. (2010). The Hands of The Living God. *Psychoanalytic Dialogues*, 20, 5, 478–503.
Felman, S. and Laub, D. (1992). *Testimony: Crises of Witnessing in Literature, Psychoanalysis, and History*. New York, NY and London, England: Routledge.
Ferris, A. (2003). The Disembodied Spirit. *The Disembodied Spirit Exhibition Catalog*, Bowdoin College Museum of Art, Brunswick, ME, 32–43.
Freud, S. (1920). Beyond the Pleasure Principle. *The Standard Edition of the Complete Psychological Works of Sigmund Freud*, Volume XVIII (1920–1922): Beyond the Pleasure Principle, Group Psychology and Other Works, 1–64
Ghent, E. (1990). Masochism, Submission, Surrender: Masochism as a Perversion of Surrender. *Contemporary Psychoanalysis*, 26, 108–136.
Gordon, A. (2008). *Ghostly Matters: Haunting and the Sociological Imagination*. Minneapolis, MN and London, England: The University of Minnesota Press.
Green, A. (1998). The Primordial Mind and the Work of the Negative. *The International Journal of Psychoanalysis*, 79, 649–665.
Hambourg, M. and Fineman, M. (2002). Avedon's Endgame. Catalogue Essay from exhibition publication *Richard Avedon: Portraits September 26, 2002–January 5, 2003*. New York, NY: Harry N. Abrams.
Harris, A. (2009). You Must Remember This. *Psychoanalytic Dialogues*, 19, 1, 2–21.
Himes, M. (Spring, 2012). The Weight of the Proper Name. *Division|Review*, 4, 15–18, American Psychological Association.
Jennings, M. W., Eiland, H., and Smith, G. (Eds.) (1999) *Walter Benjamin: Selected Writings Volume 2 1931–1934*. Cambridge, MT: The Belknap Press of Harvard University Press.
Keller, C. (2013). *Francesca Woodman 1958–1981*. New York, NY: San Francisco Museum of Modern Art with DAP Museum Catalogue,.
Kohon, G. (1999). *The Dead Mother: The Work of Andre Green*. London, England and New York, NY: Routledge.
Kraus, R. (1986). Problem sets. *Francesca Woodman: Photographic work*, 41–51. New York, NY: Wellesley College Museum and Hunter College Art Gallery.
LaCapra, D. (2001). *Writing History, Writing Trauma*. Baltimore, MD and London, England: The Johns Hopkins University Press.
Laplanche, J. and Pontalis, J.-B. (1967). *The Language of Psycho-Analysis*. New York, NY: W. W. Norton and Company.
Leys, R. (2000). *Trauma: A Genealogy*. Chicago, IL and London, England: The University of Chicago Press.
Levine, H. and Reed, G. (2013). The Colorless Canvas: Representation, therapeutic action and the creation of mind. In H. Levine, G. Reed, & D. Scarfone (Eds.), *Unrepresented States and the Construction of Meaning* (pp. 42–71). London: Karnac Books.
Levi-Strauss, D. (2010). After You, Dearest Photography: Reflections on the Work of Francesca Woodman. In *Francesca Woodman*. Zurich, Berlin, New York, NY: Foundation Cartier.
Lombardi, R. (2005). On the Psychoanalytic Treatment of a Psychotic Breakdown. *Psychoanalytic Quarterly*, 74, 1069–1099.

Mantel, H. (2009). *Wolf Hall*. New York, NY: Henry Holt and Company, LLC.
McGleughlin, J. (2011). The Analyst's Necessary Vertigo. *Psychoanalytic Dialogues*, 21, 5, 630–642.
Melville, H. (1851). *Moby Dick*. New York, NY: Penguin Group; Reprint edition (1992).
Michaels, W. B. (1996). "'You who never was there': Slavery and the New Historicism, Deconstruction and the Holocaust." *Narrative*, 4(1): 1–8.
Naiburg, S. (in press). *Structure and Spontaneity in Clinical Prose: A Writer's Guide for Psychoanalysts and Psychotherapists*. New York, NY: Routledge.
Nguyen, L. (2012). Psychoanalytic activism. *Psychoanalytic Dialogues*, 29, 3, 308–317.
Ogden, T. H. (Ed.) (2001). *Conversations at the Frontier of Dreaming*. Northvale, NJ: Aronson.
Phelan, P. (2002). Francesca Woodman's photography: Death and the image one more time. *Signs: Journal of Woman in Culture and Society*, 27, 979–1004.
Pontalis, J. B. (1999). *Perdre De Vue*. Paris, France: Gallimard.
Raymond, C. (2010). *Francesca Woodman and the Kantian Sublime*. Surrey, England and Burlington, VT: Ashgate Publishing.
Reis, B. (2009). Performative and Enactive Features of Psychoanalytic Witnessing: The Transference as the Scene of Address. *The International Journal of Psychoanalysis*, 90, 1359–1372.
Seligman, S. (2007). Mentalization and Metaphor, Acknowledgment and Grief: Forms of Transformation in the Reflective Space. *Psychoanalytic Dialogues*, 17, 321–344.
Slavin, M. (2011). Lullaby on the Dark Side: Existential Anxiety, Meaning Making, and the Dialectics of Self and Other. In L. Aron & A. Harris (Eds.), *Relational Psychoanalysis* (Vol. I). Hillsdale, NJ: The Analytic Press.
Solomon-Godeau, A. (1986). Just Like a Woman. *Francesca Woodman: Photographic work*, 11–37. New York, NY: Wellesley College Museum and Hunter College Art Gallery.
Stern, D. B. (1983). Unformulated Experience—From Familiar Chaos to Creative Disorder. *Contemporary Psychoanalysis*, 19, 1–9.
Stern, D. B. (1985). Psychoanalysis and Truth: Current issues (A Symposium)—Introduction to Some Controversies Regarding Constructivism and Psychoanalysis. *Contemporary Psychoanalysis*, 21, 201–207.
Stern, D. B. (1989). The Analyst's Unformulated Experience of the Patient. *Contemporary Psychoanalysis*, 25(1), 1–33.
Stern, D. B. (1997). *Unformulated Experience: From Dissociation to Imagination in Psychoanalysis*. Hillsdale, NJ: The Analytic Press.
Stern, D. N., Sander, L. W., Nahum, J. P., Harrison, A. M., Lyons-Ruth, K., Morgan, A. C., Bruschweilerstern, N., and Tronick, E. Z. (1998). Non-Interpretive Mechanisms in Psychoanalytic Therapy: The 'Something More' Than Interpretation. *Int. J. Psycho-Anal.*, 79: 903–921.
Stolorow, R. D., Brandchaft, B., and Atwood, G. E. (1987). *Psychoanalytic Treatment: An Intersubjective Approach*. Hillsdale, NJ: The Analytic Press.
Stolorow, R. (2007). *Trauma and Human Existence: Autobiographical, Psychoanalytic, and Philosophical Reflections*. New York, NY and London, England: Routledge.
St. Vincent Millay, E. (1917). *Renaissance and other Poems*. New York, NY: Harper.
Sundell, M. (2003). Francesca Woodman Reconsidered: A Conversation with George Baker, Ann Daly, Nancy Davenport, Laura Larson and Margaret Sundell. *Art Journal*, 62, 2: 53–67.

Townsend, C. (2006). Scattered in Space and Time. *Francesca Woodman.* Oxford: Phaidon. 6–71.
Willis, S. (2010). *The Woodmans* [documentary film]. C. Scott Films LLC.
Winnicott, D.W. (1969). The Use of an Object. *International Journal of Psycho-Analysis*, 50, 711–716.
Winterson, J. (2011). *Why Be Happy When You Could Be Normal?* New York, NY: Grove Press.
Woodman, F. (1981). *Some Disordered Interior Geometries.* Philadelphia, PA: Synapse Press.
Woodman, F. (2006). Seething with Ideas. *Francesca Woodman.* Oxford: Phaidon, 240–5.

Community & culture

Chapter 6

The past is the presence between us

Psychoanalysis and the specter of the Shoah

Emily A. Kuriloff

It was 1960s America, but the talk at my family's dinner table was as much about Nazi collaborators, righteous gentiles, and family members I had never met as it was about the wars in Vietnam or Israel. The famous and the infamous, and my relatives whose fate had rested in their hands, haunted us.

Yet, as an adult psychologist in the late 1980s, I tended to view the Shoah as a prop in a more universal drama. While my family history might determine the content, even the degree of my preoccupation, Nazis were to be viewed as a metaphor for more essential conflicts surrounding internal drives, for instance.

It is not that this understanding was incorrect, but that it is incomplete. My training as an interpersonal/relational psychoanalyst gradually taught me to consider both the predilection of the individual, his or her social context, and the accidents of fate in determining a life. In this spirit the iconic dinners of my childhood returned to me. As I began to appreciate their particular influence, I thought not only of my family, but of my professional "family" as well—the mostly Jewish European psychoanalysts who were also caught in the scourge of the Nazi era. What effect, I wondered, did their personal histories have upon their work, and thus the direction of the psychoanalytic traditions that I—that my generation—have inherited? This query culminated in the volume *Contemporary Psychoanalysis and the Legacy of the Third Reich* (2014), an attempt to historicize an intellectual and clinical tradition, relying heavily on interviews with analyst émigrés/survivors and/or scholars of the period, thus evoking the "ghosts" of an auspicious, terrific past. It is indeed this past, in many of the interviews, that is the presence between us.

However, contextualizing meaning in this way threatens to become its own version of Truth, neglecting, ironically, the dynamic quality of context—both past and present—that honors individual subjectivity. Thus while some (Aron and Starr, 2013; Boyarin, 1997) stress the impact of European Anti-semitism on a psychoanalytic sensibility that jettisons its Jewish roots and sensibility, Erich Fromm, who trained at the Berlin Psychoanalytic Institute, did not jettison his Jewish roots, nor did he feel particularly touched by anti-Semitism in pre-war Germany (Friedman, 2013, p.51). Indeed, Fromm felt comfortable studying Transference and Countertransference, but also Torah and Talmud in Berlin. If there are moral skeins in Fromm's theories and technique, these may reflect both his psychoanalytic and ecclesiastic influences. Thus, after Hitler became chancellor of Germany, Fromm wrote his book, *Escape From Freedom* (1941), in which he presented Nazism's success as indicative of the individual's tendency to succumb to the group for fear of loss of love or disapprobation. Here Fromm revises Freud's 1923 conflict theory— originally conceived as the chafing of internal, forbidden wishes against guilt and fear of punishment—to include that between self and society.

Fromm's Jewish moral and ethical compass bumps up against the outside culture, leaving the individual to choose his or her path despite the external pressure. In a section of the *Mishnah,* or Jewish recorded oral Law, entitled, "Ethics of the Fathers" (Perkei Avot), Hillel is quoted as saying, "If I am not for myself, who will be for me?" Another Rabbi advises, "In a place where there are no men, strive to be a man." How similar these pronouncements sound to Fromm's model of the healthy individual—embracing, rather than escaping his or her freedom to choose the righteous path, despite the pressure of the moment.

Fromm's unique view of conflict was applied to a world stage on which the survival of civilization hung in the balance. This focus, however relevant to the moment, also "haunts" the overall quality of Fromm's thinking for the rest of his days. Even as he introduced a useful revision to Freudian conflict theory, he ironically left the reader and the patient little room for conflict. The ghosts of external oppression and cruelty are the backdrop, so that there can only be a decision to go in the more morally righteous direction as opposed to the considerably less righteous, less "Jewish" decision to surrender to the mindless mob. When Fromm put this so- called choice to his patients, they could well feel, according to one supervisee and colleague, as if they are being "cracked over the head with a stick" (Maccoby, 1990, p. 65). If Fromm's' psychoanalytic sensibility also helped him to appreciate the presence of a gray area—the struggle back and forth that is itself transformative, or the mourning for what is always lost by virtue of one's having chosen—such a view did not cancel out his Rabbinic affinity for ethical imperatives amidst the ghouls of the Shoah.

On the other hand, the Viennese psychoanalyst Ernst Kris, born a Jew, was so assimilated into German high kultur that his son, the analyst Anton Kris comments, "If there was any God in our house . . . it was Goethe" (Kuriloff, 2014, p. 12). Conflict for Kris was intrapsychic and universal, fueling his theory of mind and therapeutic action essentially unaltered by culture and circumstance, reflecting his secular focus on science, free from the subjectivity of spirituality. Was this Kris's deliberate rejection of Judaism? Was Kris motivated to eschew his identity in order to buttress his masculinity? According to A. Kris, religion was never important to his father, nor was he educated in Jewish law or tradition. His identity, therefore, neither felt to him to be under attack, nor in need of revision. The psychoanalytically trained historian Thomas Kohut, speaks about *his* father, Heinz Kohut, in similar terms:

> More than anything, my father was deeply and profoundly Viennese. He regularly extolled the riches of the capital city—its art, music, literature. He visited the landmark Austrian novelist, Robert Musil, author of *The Man Without Qualities*, bringing the surprised author a bouquet of flowers, for instance.
>
> (Kuriloff, 2014)

The elder Kohut was in fact raised as a cosmopolitan, a product of a classical European gymnasiaum and university education. Thomas Kohut thus objects to the idea put forth by Blum (Kuriloff, 2014, p. 12) that Kohut disavowed a Jewish identity because he was concerned about rumors that he was homosexual, and notions that Jewish men, as earlier noted, were effeminate. Heinz Kohut's biographer, Charles Strozier (2007), also suggests that Kohut actively denied his Jewishness for this, and other reasons, to which Thomas Kohut replies:

> [Strozier's] accusation that my father was lying, or being deliberately misleading about who he was, represents a failure to understand what it meant to be Jewish in Vienna in the decades before the Nazi

Anschluss, or to appreciate the deep psychological wounds inflicted by anti-Semitic persecution and flight. Indeed, those who insist that people who are 'racially Jewish' must either identify themselves as Jewish or be dismissed as 'self denying' or 'self hating' Jews are essentializing Jewishness in profoundly troubling, indeed racial, ways.

(Kuriloff, 2014, p. 12)

Imagine, then, the compound trauma for Kohut and others like him, long esteemed within a pluralistic milieu, suddenly expelled on fear of death precisely because of such bizarrely essentialist and racial notions.

As we consider the impact of the specter of the Shoah among Jewish psychoanalysts, therefore, we cannot make out any linear, nor certainly any single narrative. We must proceed in the quintessentially psychoanalytic realm of subjective experience, as hard to reify as the tenuous apparitions that nonetheless make their presence known in ways particular to each haunted soul.

Thomas Kohut, once again, claims that it was in fact his father's abrupt loss of his *secular* identity that haunted him. "One of the two greatest narcissistic injuries of his life was being cast out for being labelled Jewish," the other being his father's battle with the cancer that precipitated his untimely death. "On one of our two trips back to Austria," Thomas Kohut continued:

> We were hiking in the mountains and met some people from the area, with whom my father easily spoke an Austrian German. I suddenly saw a different, much less tense, more animated part of my father as he conversed with these people. It was only then that I realized all that my father had lost and missed, that the man I knew was more con-stricted, that he had only been engaging a part of himself.
>
> (Kuriloff, 2014, p.13)

Like so many of the émigrés I have encountered in my research, Heinz Kohut's past injury insidiously occupied his present. His son reports that he "never bought property in America," for instance, fearing the next expulsion. "There was even a time, when George Wallace [the racist governor of Alabama in the 1960s] looked like a viable presidential candidate, and my father was seriously thinking that things might eventually come to pass that we might have to flee the United States" (p. 13).

Indeed, Heinz Kohut responded to a journalist's question regarding his interest in narcissism by referring to his own expulsion from Vienna in 1938: "I've led two totally different, perhaps unbridgeable lives." It was this, he elaborated, that made him alert to "the problem of the fragmented self" (Cited in Quinn, 1984, p. 124) suggests a link between his ordeal and his emphasis on a cohesive sense of self as a developmental progression distinct from energic, dynamic considerations, a shift that revolutionized all of psychoanalytic theory and practice.

Trauma, so difficult to mentalize and integrate, thus occupies the liminal space between past and present, between private and professional life, hanging about elusively, and yet full with complexity and contradiction within and between one individual and the next. Sometimes the past has a felicitious effect, such as Kohut's discoveries regarding the fragmented self, or Fromm's notions of individual agency against mass movements driven by base aims. In other instances specters obscure or blot out the light, and can account for blind spots that persist. Kestenberg & Kestenberg (1982) for example, note that Kohut and many other prominent analyst émigrés neglected the role of trauma in their clinical work. Among their many examples, Kestenberg & Kestenberg refer to Kohut's case of Mr. A., whose childhood was interrupted by Nazi persecution, and whose symptoms quite obviously reflect this trauma. Yet Kohut denied any connection between this history and the patient's difficulties, and focused instead on pre-Oedipal pathology.

Psychoanalytic theory does posit that it is one's early life, including infantile fantasy, that has the sizable effect on both the quality and the degree of one's response to later trauma. Still, the overall neglect of Holocaust trauma in patients' material, well documented by Bergmann and Jacovy (1982), is something else again. One might consider that in some cases, such neglect of an experience that helped define a century, let alone the lives of so many of the leading theoreticians and clinicians in the field, represents a repetition of the unattended-to trauma, this time in a large-scale psychic exile. What do I mean by this? In such professional discourse, an authority (the analyst) marginalizes the émigré or survivor's experience, who must abandon the past (more or less dissociate and/or repress) and "adapt"—a term with the Ego Psychologists were quite familiar—to this psychoanalytic culture.

To complicate matters further, individuals who study the era—including some émigrés—interpret its impact based upon their subjectivity, their singular experience. Take, for example, the premature end to Otto Fenichel. Historian Russell Jacoby (1983) describes how Fenichel, having fled Europe as much because of his leftist politics as his Jewishness, felt compelled to repeat his clinical training in the USA in order to become license eligible, rather than risk being viewed as a "second class citizen" (p. 131), a fate he feared would befall him in any prominent analytic organization in post-war America. According to Jacoby, Fenichel literally worked himself to death, succumbing during a difficult internship intended for beginning students less than half his age. Jacoby tells the story in this way to bolster his conviction that American "professionalization" and "medicalization" transformed psychoanalysis by rendering its ideas in a "dry scientific idiom." This psychoanalysis was no longer the European effort marked by "intellectual fervor, reforming zeal, and theoretical boldness" (p. 142) that it had once been. If "political Freudians" continued to critique theory and culture at all, they did so in private, in a *Rundbrief,* a newsletter passed among them in secret. Never again did they publish or publicly present such politicized, socially progressive material.

Jacoby (1983) reminds us that Fenichel had been known in Europe as one of the "political Freudians," a group that included such personages as Edith Jacobson and Wilhelm Reich. According to Jacoby, emigration to moderate capitalist democracies inhibited Fenichel and others from expanding on their work in exile, or continuing the critique of culture and society that had characterized their ideas in Europe. Their earlier views regarding sexuality, Jacoby stresses, had an impact on child rearing and education, for example. Such a focus is not evident after emigration. Apparently spooked by Nazi totalitiarianism, their silence only grew during the actual presence of Joe McCarthy. In fact, Jacoby characterizes Fenichel's tome, *The Psychoanalytic Theory of Neurosis,* published after his escape from fascism, less as an attempt to salvage the European psychoanalytic tradition than as a capitulation to the mainstream American conservatism, embraced by the medical establishment. He criticizes the book as mechanical, even perfunctory. However, this dismal picture may not be the entire, or even the accurate story.

That is, Ernst Kris's son, the analyst Anton Kris, has his own private memories that counter what he refers to as "the Jacoby hypothesis on Fenichel," (Kuriloff, 2014, p. 41). A. Kris disagrees with the premise that Fenichel was beleaguered, intimated, and ultimately defeated by his European expulsion and the trials of re-establishing himself in a conservative, even reactionary post-war America. "Fenichel died of a Berry brain aneurysm, which is a congenital [rather than a stress induced] condition," Kris continued, "In fact we saw him just before he died and he was quite well."

In a presentation at an international conference in Tel Aviv, Seth Aronson (2009), also challenged the notion that the European émigrés completely lost their "cutting edge" and became more conservative and compliant after their expulsion by the Third Reich. Aronson focuses upon the Berlin born analyst, Edith Jacobson, herself imprisoned by Hitler in the 1930s because of her status as one of the "political Freudians," suspected of having knowledge of Leftist activities among her patients. Despite her life-altering trauma, Aronson argues that Jacobson's post-war innovations were indeed revolutionary—particularly her linking intrapsychic life to the quality of early relationships. Her stance, Aronson argues, was true to her radical zeal, particularly because she ran the risk of being marginalized by the dominant émigré Ego Psychologists, who, having also escaped Hitler's grasp, positioned themselves as the only true heirs to Freud.

Clearly, then, various attempts to historicize psychoanalysis in the context of the shadow of history often conflict with one another, in as much as individual subjectivity is never uniform. Still, they capture a piece of the truth without being unconditionally or universally valid, and taken together provide some narrative meaning to what has been intimated.

As the beginning of this chapter implies, my perceptions are also inevitably tinged with elusive, yet recurrent specters from *my* past. Among other things, I cannot exclude the fact that I am the scion of the still ever-present grandmother of my childhood. The official tale of her life juxtaposed an impoverished, anti-Semitic Poland with what she called "La Belle France," where her parents moved their young family because there were fewer restrictions for Jews in Paris. That this same nation later transported her brothers and sister, along with thousands of others, from the French-run transit camp at Drancy to their deaths in Auschwitz was apparently never considered side by side with the beginning of the story. In fact, it appeared as though America—the nation that actually protected my grandmother—was at fault, never as good as France. Thus she required shipments of croissants, brioches, crème fraiche, and Camembert from friends and family to make up for the "abysmal" products in the United States. She criticized American art and music as lowbrow and judged the comfortable life around her as typically American—empty and materialistic.

Yet there were clues to a less than idyllic past. She refused to allow me to leave her side when we were out in public and panicked if she lost sight of me for even a moment. Her psychosomatic symptoms made her a fixture in the local emergency room. It seems to me now that my grandmother could neither accept nor relinquish the great love and murderous hate that formed the arc of her life. Thus she could not know or speak of her history fully—instead it was enacted in the present. My grandmother behaved as if nothing had been taken and at the same time she clung too tightly to what was indeed gone, as a means both to defend against and to relive the terror of losing again and again.

As might be expected, my grandmother's ghosts ineffably became my mother's, and then mine. The Weimar constitution in Germany before 1933, its freedoms greater even than those granted citizens of the United States at the time, and Leon Blum's socialist France, where a Jew could emerge from the shadows to create a just world for all, do not feel like historical documents or events to me. Instead, they are omens, and warn of the terrifyingly swift and tragic doom that is perpetually to follow. As the Egyptian Jewish writer Andre Aciman (1999) puts it, "An exile reads change the way he reads time, memory, self, love, fear, beauty: in the key of loss" (p. 22). My grandmother's lost European world is sufficiently similar, at a distance, to the one in which psychoanalysis was born and its hopes nurtured and destroyed. My study of the analyst émigrés and survivors thus threatens to become her story and, by extension, my own. I must take pains to listen to the psychoanalytic words and ideas for other, less self-referential meanings, and must learn to employ perhaps more complex notions not yet formulated. The challenge of this inquiry is thus simultaneously historical, analytic, and self-analytic (Kuriloff, 2014, p. 17).

Such self reflexivity is both provoked and avoided in relation. Consider here my conversations with the German psychoanalyst Regine Lockot, internationally recognized expert on the history of her profession in Germany. When I sought her guidance as part of my research for my book, she invited me to Berlin so I might participate in a session of her forum, a discussion group of fellow professionals interested in the topic of analysis before, during, and after the Third Reich.

Lockot, whose definitive volumes on the subject (1985, 1994) have not yet been translated into English, was born in 1946, after the war. She credits her own early experiences as contributing to her writing. At school she became quite close to a teacher whom she refers to as a mentor—a woman who broadened her otherwise narrow exposure to the world. Only later did she discover that this Jewish woman had been interned at Terezin concentration camp in what is now the Czech Republic.

Warmly welcomed into her West Berlin office with homemade Christmas cookies, Lockot and her colleagues first asked about my experience of their city. I began by noting the many commemorative monuments to Nazi victims. We shared our admiration for Daniel Liebeskind's brilliant architecture of the Jewish Museum—his uneven walkways, a staircase leading nowhere, the engulfing Holocaust "tower." But then Lockot added poignantly, "They should have kept it empty." Feeling understood, I shared my sense that the museum's exhibits objectify Jews and Jewishness as extinct artifacts of the past. Then I went further, remarking "Hitler got his wish—he had been saving religious articles in Prague, hoping to create a museum for a 'Judenrein' world." After an awkward pause, someone said, "That is the strongest indictment I have yet heard of the place" (Kuriloff, 2014, p. 8).

My words reflected my conflict about sitting among open minded and welcoming German colleagues in what felt like a particularly lively, twenty-first century European capitol. I had spent the day in the old Jewish neighborhood of East Berlin, where I found so many small bronze plaques embedded into the gray cobblestoned streets, all indicating where a Jew had once lived. A name, when and where he or she was murdered ("*emordet*") is engraved on each one. Families are clustered together.

I began to search for these stones everywhere I walked, appreciating the chance to honor the lost. Such public signs, however, did not banish the my private ghosts, particularly at certain moments; when I noted that the centrally located memorial—monoliths that commemorated the "Murdered Jews of Europe"—was built along Hannah Arendt Strasse, renamed for the philosopher whose controversial book (1963) suggested that a passive European Jewish community was complicit in the final solution, augmenting their own genocide; when I encountered a drunken, brazen flirt who was wearing a tee-shirt upon which the term *Aryan* was printed in gothic lettering. This, despite being told that it is officially illegal to display the swastika or utter any Nazi epithet. (Does Aryan count?) I'd been replaced not by a mediating, integrating Ego, but by the threat of punishment—the Superego. Little chance, I fretted as I heard about these laws and later as I read the tee-shirt, for greater self awareness, for urges tolerated rather than enacted in a less brittle, and more self reflexive way.

Regine Lockot listened intently to my concerns, and also had much to say about her city Berlin. In addition to her historical acumen, Lockot was generous with her feelings and stories, helping to create what she aptly terms a "private space" for testimony and witnessing. Elaborating on the silence of the German analysts in the first decades after the war regarding the fate of their Jewish colleagues, she shared the roots of her involvement in the research (personal interview, 2010):

> For me, when I started to be interested after the war, there was more to it than shame, guilt, or avoidance. I did not feel able, as a non-Jew, to engage this, as if I had no right, it was not fair of me—it was not my story. When I started my research, I felt I needed to clear up what happened in Germany among the Germans first.
> (Kuriloff, 2014, p. 82)

Later, when she moved on to interviewing Jewish analysts, her youthful enthusiasm was not matched by adequate sensitivity, and she shared moments with me in great detail, as if they had happened to her only yesterday, as if they remained, at her side:

> I had some contact with Anna Freud—I had an appointment with her in London but it was cancelled because it was the same day that Dorothy Burlingham died. Since I had time, I contacted Paula Heimann instead. She asked me to send written questions... But I was naïve, and lacked awareness... I asked inappropriate questions... For instance, I asked about analysts' involvement in the early Nazi Euthanasia project. To this Heimann replied to me something like, "Its too much to explain," adding, "If you want to get back your ques-tions, please send postage..."
> (Kuriloff, 2014, p. 83)

Lockot feels that over the years she has come to better appreciate the deeply personal and complex feelings of all involved.

I was impressed by Lockot's openness regarding these struggles. Her disclosures helped me to acknowledge my own difficulties, particularly when she questioned my automatic assumption that second- or third-hand interpretations of data were based on fact. Indeed, in her later edits to the manuscript of my book, she regretted that I could not read German, for then I would have sensed the tone and content of the long unavailable eyewitness accounts she uncovered during the 1980s. She wanted me to glean a "special feeling" for what happens to people when "horror has been dealt as if it is the most normal thing in the world, and normality is made horrifying" (Kuriloff, 2014, p. 83).

When I subsequently presented this interview material at a conference at the William Alanson White Institute in New York, psychologist and then analytic candidate Katarina Rothe (personal interview, 2012) had some additional interpretations based on her own research (2009, 2012) on post-war anti-Semitism in Germany. A former assistant professor at the University of Leipzig, Rothe explored contemporary attitudes towards the Shoah via interviews with non-Jewish Germans. When she reviewed the transcripts of these discussions, she detected unmentalized enactments between herself and her subjects. Including her own subjectivity as part of her data, she reckoned that she and the interviewees had repeatedly oscillated between the roles of victim and victimizer. Employing the psychoanalytic language of Melanie Klein, Rothe concluded from her data that "projective identification"—the placing of unwanted, unbearable affects in the other—becomes the prototype for relatedness between generations of Germans when they encounter the specter of National Socialism.

At my invitation, Rothe applied her researcher's ear to the record of interactions between myself and Lockot, and found evidence that the two of us were also projecting and playing out history. Was Lockot unconsciously enacting a role reversal when she spoke of her fellow Germans' horrifying experiences, Rothe pondered? Who, Rothe continued, was actually the victim of horror, Jew or German? Yet, even as she shared her thoughts, Rothe stopped herself midsentence in order to observe that now she, a non-German Jew, was becoming Lockot's accuser, a recursive pattern in lieu of mentalizing the identifications. Yet again the ghosts of the past occupy us, including their cruelty and destruction. She told me flatly, "I only became aware of my latent accuser position in the course of doing my study," and moreover that "I only became aware of this personal defense against the transmitted shame and projected 'guilt' feeling in my own family even later." Such "transmitted shame and projected guilt" referred to the fact that Rothe researched and discovered that her grandfather, previously idealized in the family as a brave, fallen soldier, was instead an avowed National Socialist (p. 84).

Refusing to hold herself above the fray, Rothe continued to examine my conversation with Lockot. The "special feeling" to which Lockot referred, seemingly unavailable to me because of my inability to read German, reminded Rothe of the "phantasm" of the anointed German people during the Nazi scourge—the *volksmeinschaft*. This, she explained, was the genetically superior and innately special group to which the inferior *undermenchen*, the Jews, could never belong. At this moment I added, "And that is the way I think of Jews when I talk to Germans sometimes—as special, elevated martyrs, because of their suffering at the hands of the inferior, bestial German Huns—all of whom are dead, but very much alive to me" (p. 84). There we were for a moment, our family's pasts hanging around in our presence, which also, surprisingly, prompted a moment of meeting between us, a Jewish grand-niece of Shoah victims, and the non-Jewish granddaughter of a Nazi.

There were also such moments between myself and Lockot. At one point she had told me a personal story concerning the site of the Wanasee conference, a suburban Berlin villa, where top SS officers had decided the "Final Solution to the Jewish Problem." The villa is now a national museum:

> I saw the exhibits [at the villa]—some photos in which Nazis are smiling and laughing as they taunt and humiliate Jews. These disturbed me very much. And I thought, "This is sadistic pleasure."
>
> (Kuriloff, 2014, p. 84)

We wondered together what helps or hinders the individual from becoming compulsively sadistic, at the expense of other modulating feelings and awareness. I noted that some non- Jewish analysts who stayed on at the reconfigured Berlin institute during the Third Reich seemed to more or less turn a blind eye to the horror in their midst, and others embraced at least parts of Hitler's aims. This, despite their having been psychoanalysed, often by Freud's closest associates. Then I noted a comment made by the French Jewish analyst, Janine Chasseguet-Smirgel (1988), who claimed that in order to prevent such passivity, avoidance, or even capitulation to evil, we all must recognize the "Hitler in us" (p. 1061), for he, and those before him, linger still.

Lockot and I also wondered if it were only an inherent, or learned sadomasochism that undermines the capacity for self-reflection and responsibility. The earlier noted historian and psychoanalyst Thomas Kohut

(2012), in his deconstruction of transcripts of post-war interviews with enthusiastic National Socialists after the war, suggests that more is afoot. Contrary to the German analysts Alexander and Margarete Mitscherlich's (1975) thesis that excessive guilt renders post-Nazi Germans unable to mourn, Kohut instead posits the opposite: Mourning must proceed a capacity to feel guilt and responsibility. Kohut notes the pride and optimism in the accounts of former party members, and views the enthusiasm as a means to avoid the experiences of defeat concerning what happened before, during, and after the war. Kohut posits further that if loss is consciously denied, disavowed, or split off, so too must be the defensive, destructive responses being used as a counterweight. Put differently, accepting their murderousness may require that Germans understand its roots in narcissistic injury.

On a snowy night in Berlin, Lockot and I struggled with the many shadows of our pasts, and grappled with one another. Who, and in what combination or degree were European psychoanalysts like the two of us—more or less afflicted with sadism, driven by narcissism, haunted by guilt, shame, grief, and a sense of both vulnerability and self righteousness? How has Berlin's psychoanalytic history, the horror that occurred at the former jewel in Freud's crown, affected our views of the mind, of motivation?

Among these themes, I shared with Lockot that battles regarding both Freudian and Kleinian notions of a "Death Drive." I shared my findings that acceptance of such a drive varied based upon whether or not analysts were Jewish, or non-Jewish, native, or émigré analysts forced to leave their homelands. Paradoxically, and perhaps defensively or even dissociatively, émigré/Jewish analysts were less likely to accept an immutable destructiveness, despite their personal proximity to the human behavior known collectively as the Shoah (see also Chapter Three of my book, in which the Freud-Klein "Controversial discussions' in London during the Blitz are addressed along these lines).

Ultimately, there is enough evidence to conclude that psychoanalytic ideas and traditions conceived and practiced by European Jewish founders and followers were, and continue to be visited by ghosts of the Shoah. Most of our foremothers and fathers, those whose homelands and families were transformed by catastrophe, cannot talk with us, even as they linger amongst us. Indeed, the absence of an actual dialogue with them does not cancel out their presence and the presence of their trauma, but neither can we presume, generalize, nor, more pointedly, reify our ghosts from a most extraordinary time.

This chapter is an adaptation of Emily Kuriloff's book *Contemporary Psychoanalysis and the Legacy of the Third Reich: History, Memory, Tradition*, Routledge, 2013, with permission from Taylor & Francis, LLC.

Bibliography

Aciman, A. (1999). Shadow Cities. In A. Aciman (Ed.), *Letters of Transit: Reflections on Exile, Identity, Language and Loss* (pp. 15–35). New York. NY: New Press.

Aron, L. (2006). Reflections on Heinz Kohut's Religious Identity and Anti-Semitism: Discussion of C. Strozier's "Heinz Kohut and the Meanings of Identity." *Contemporary Psychoanalysis*, 43(2), 411–420.

Aron, L. and Starr, K. (2013). *A Psychotherapy for the People*. New York, NY and London: Routledge.

Aronson, S. (2009). *The Postwar Politics of Edith Jacobson*. Presented at International Association of Relational Psychoanalysis and Psychotherapy Conference on Trauma and Memory, June, Tel Aviv, Israel.

Arendt, H. (1963). *Eichmann in Jerusalem: A Report on the Banality of Evil*. New York, NY and London: Penguin.

Bergman, M and Jacovy, M. (1982). *Generations of the Holocaust*. New York, NY: Columbia University Press.

Boyarin, D. (1997). *Unheroic Conduct: The Rise of Heterosexuality and the Invention of the Jewish Ma*n. Berkeley, CA: University of California Press.

Chasseguet-Smirgel, J. (1988). Review of J-L. Evard (Ed.) Les Années Brunes. Psychoanalysis under the Third Reich. *Journal of the American Psychoanalytic Association*, 36(3), 1059–1066.

Friedman, L. (2013). *The Lives of Erich Fromm: Love's Prophet*. New York, NY: Columbia University Press.

Fromm, E. (1941). *Escape from Freedom*. New York, NY: Farrar Strauss.

Fromm, E. (1968). *Thoughts on Politics*. Unpublished manuscript, Fromm Archives, Werner Funk, executor.

Jacoby, R. (1983). *The Repression of Psychoanalysis: Otto Fenichel and the Political Freudians*. New York, NY: Basic Books.

Kestenberg, J. and Kestenberg, M. (1982). The Background of the Study. In M. Bergman and M. Jacovy (Eds.), *Generations of the Holocaust* (pp. 33–45). New York, NY: Columbia University Press.

Kohut, T. (2012). *A German Generation. An Experiential History of the Twentieth Century*. New Haven, CT: Yale University Press.

Kris, E. (1975). *The Selected Papers of Ernst Kris*. New Haven, CT and London: Yale University Press.

Kuriloff, E. (2014). *Contemporary Psychoanalysis and the Legacy of the Third Reich. History, Memory, Tradition*. New York, NY and London: Routledge.

Lockot, R. (1985). *Erinnern und Durcharbeiten: Aur Geschichte der Psychoanlyse und Psychotherapie im Nationalsozialismus*. [Remembering and Working Through: On the History of Psychoanalysis and Psychotherapy in National Socialism.] Frankfort Am Main: Fisher Taschenbuch.

Lockot, R. (1994). *Die Reinigung der Psychoanalyse. Die Deutsche Psychoanalystische Gesellschaft im Spiegel von Dokumenten und Zeitzeugen*. (1933–1951). [The Cleansing of Psychoanalysis. The German Psychoanalytic Society as reflected in Documents and by Witnesses to History. (1933–1951)]. Tubingen: Edition Diskord.

Maccoby, M. (1990). Erich Fromm's Contribution to Psychoanalysis. In M. Cortina and M. Maccoby (Eds.), *A Prophetic Analyst* (pp. 61–91). Northvale, NJ: Jason Aronson Inc.

Mitsherlich, A. and Mitsherlich, M. (1975). *The Inability to Mourn: Principles of Collective Behavior*. New York, NY: Random House.

Quinn, S. (1984). Psychoanalysis and the Holocaust: A Roundtable. In S. Luel and P. Marcus (Eds.), *Psychoanalytic Reflections on the Holocaust: Selected Essays* (pp. 209–229). New York, NY: Ktav.

Rothe, K. (2009). *Das (Nicht-)Sprechen über die Judenvernichtung. Psychische Weiterwirkungen des Holocaust in mehreren Generationen nicht-jüdischer Deutscher*. [(Non) Speaking about the Extermination of the Jews. Psychical Aftermaths of the Holocaust in Several Generations of non-Jewish Germans]. Gießen: Psychosozial-Verlag.

Rothe, K. (2012). Anti-Semitism in Germany today and the Intergenerational Transmission of Guilt and Shame. *Psychoanalysis, Culture & Society,* 17(1), 16–34.

Strozier, C. (2001). *Heinz Kohut: The Making of a Psychoanalyst*. New York, NY: FarrarStrauss Giroux.

Strozier, C. (2007). Heinz Kohut and the Meaning of Identity. *Contemporary Psychoanalysis*, 43(3), 399–411.

Chapter 7

Ghosts and the sexual boundary violation

The limits of an idea

Muriel Dimen

In the intimate sphere, the ghostly carries a certain heft. In the public domain, not so much. A metaphor goes only so far.

Intimate

The sexual boundary violation that came my way was, like any self-respecting golem, inanimate, amorphous, an anthropomorphic figure of rock and clay. A haint, it ghosted me, I see now. I was unaware of it, though. All I had was petrified knowledge.

It's not that I didn't try to speak. But even when I described the injury to my women's group, it remained a story made of wood. I confided in a Zen priest, who, moved, wrote a poem about me telling him. I told my second analyst, but did not feel that my bewilderment made an imprint. I kept trying to spill the beans, I see now. But the thing had no voice.

It did not speak until writing made it alive.

There is a step between writing and life though, at least in this case: listening. Or rather seeing. Or perhaps synesthesia. A witness who, hearing me, discerned the eeriness I lived with. Someone who could sense the lost soul in the golem.

The golem had to become a ghost. Not a thing in the darkness but a message from the past that could be read and re-read, its meaning emergent, legible only when the elixir of close attention falls on the invisible ink in which it is written.

I do not really know how I came to know I could speak. Once again I can recount the sequence of events. But the emotional process remains illegible.

*

By the same token, I don't know how much I should speak here. Think of it as ghosts interfering with me. Having recounted the sexual boundary violation that I was subject of and to (Dimen, 2011), I wonder whether I ought repeat it here. Will I bore my readers with (what may seem) a stale saga? For those who have not read that original essay and/or heard me speak of the events at various venues, will I be saying too little? providing insufficient context? Perhaps you will hear me as too attached to the secondary gains of victimhood. Perhaps you will think I am self-centered. Perhaps I am.

I can't figure it out. So I will proceed as I did in the first place when I decided to speak: Just do it.

In 1968, at the age of 26 and a graduate student in another field and mostly illiterate in psychoanalytic process and history, I entered treatment with an impeccably credentialed psychoanalyst. Five years later, I was an assistant professor about to attend an annual conference and set on sleeping with a man I'd met the previous year. Off and on, I'd been sharing my exciting, guilty plan with Dr. O. Though I'd often discussed sex, I see, looking back, that this was the first time I owned my sexual intentionality.

The session ended, Dr. O walked me to the door, I said, "I'm scared, I want a hug." (This was not the first hug: when, after I'd sat up on the couch at another session's end, I was weeping about my father's death the previous year, Dr. O had sat next to me and put his arm around my shoulders.) As I was ending this embrace, I kissed his cheek; I don't think there'd been a kiss before. And then he said, and this was a definite first—and last—"No, how about a real kiss?" So—it wasn't even a question, because, as the quip goes, there's a "trance" in "transference"—I kissed his mouth. He returned the favor with his tongue—at which point, I recall a feeling of shock, and then a feeling of ignoring the shock. He chuckled: "Oops, I'm getting a hard-on, I better stop." In me, nothing or, rather, awareness of nothing. Call it a confusion of tongues.

I left, went to the conference, had disappointing intercourse, never saw the guy again, returned to analysis, did not speak of hug or hard-on or French kiss, and never did anything like it again in a treatment that lasted for seven more years. Dr. O did not mention it either.

*

For years, I wanted to write about this most peculiar sexual encounter with my first analyst, but could never find the first line. Ghosts of past, present, and future obtruded everywhere. But then, 31 years later, in 2004, my opportunity arrived: An invitation to speak on a panel about infidelity and its clinical ramifications. As I was picking up the phone to decline on the grounds of lacking clinical material, the lights went on: After all, did I not have a clinical account of infidelity? Did Dr. O not violate the trust of his patient, his troth to his wife, the ethics of his profession? Did I not betray the bonds of marriage?

And so I accepted. Because speakers had to turn their papers in six weeks before the conference, however, the organizing committee knew my topic in advance: I fully expected a phone call disinviting me, but that specter wasn't to appear until the next conference (see Dimen, 2011).

I grasped my stroke of luck in the midst of two intense life passages. An overlong love affair had finally ended, leaving an unpleasant ghost in its wake. And, in the third analysis I'd begun in hopes of averting that inevitability, I was being listened to and seen in a way that had not previously graced me: I felt contained as if by a friendly ghost from so early in my preverbal past as not to count as my past at all. Hence, when the sun of good fortune finally rose, my story was ready to burst into dark flower. The passion and rupture of loss had made room for the torrents of anger, grief, and guilt.

Public I

But what if we consider also that I was bearing a story that was not mine? Certainly in my tellings I sensed the ownership I was taking. And, believe me, it was hard to do: The self-focus felt inappropriate, unprofessional. Yet I felt driven to do it. No doubt the drive was personal, a healing effected by an exorcism, a turning of the golem into a ghost so that I would no longer be haunted by the fear of fury and remorse but could live in the present with sadness from the past.

It feels equally self-aggrandizing to speculate that the force which kept me writing was also larger, or other, than me. Yet, it is a premise of this collection that presences from the past accompany us as we make our ways forward. Call it haunting. As much as we are our scars, are we not also our histories? In taking psychoanalysis in, in opening my body to Dr. O in the year I'd decided to become an analyst, did I not also open to its legacy of bads as well as goods?

The intergenerational transmission of trauma is not a one-person passage: Dr. O and I cut a fine, but entirely traditional figure: The patriarchal couple, the older, virile man and the younger, sexy woman. But we did not get there by ourselves. Each of us lived by unconscious forces, we were also conducted into this combo of enactment and acting out by heterosexuality and its cultural imperatives, compulsions, and symbols.

Authors of their lives, people are always also authored by cultural and historical forces as they engage with the world to which they are heirs. Patriarchy is particularly culpable in this instance: Dr. O summons me back into the realm of the transferential erotic just as I am about to have sex with another man. As in other sexual trangressions, this incestuous act—a combination of enactment and acting-out—created the selfsame backdrop of loss against which SBVs tend to occur.

If, in speaking of the sexual transgression, I detect the weight of a past that has become mine since that time, wasn't Dr. O, in taking advantage of an erotic windfall, bearing that past too, albeit one that I cannot imagine as a conscious presence in his mind? To be sure, this repetition of a hidden and largely unspoken analytic history was also a repetition of professional infidelity—albeit with difference, since, after all, a tongue in the mouth—or even an unfelt hard-on—is not the same as the genital encounters that have baptized many an analytic couch, like Ferenczi's treatment of and affair with his mistress' daughter (the mistress he later married with Freud's encouragement), or the sexual delinquencies of Gross and Stekel and, perhaps, Jung (Makari, 2008), and, later, Horney (Falzeder, 2005–6) and, to arrive at the now, Smith (Herman, 2012).

History passed through us that day. Lacan's Third, the Law, was absent from the room, its position occupied instead by a ghost trying to speak but lacking a voice. Or, better, listeners? And the silence that followed was of a piece with all the other silencings of all the other sexual boundary violations that preceded our sad act, all the sexual violations that are taking place in and outside the consulting room everyday right now.

Shall I emphasize that point? When you read about a sexual boundary violation, it has already happened: You read about something in the past. But violations of sexual ethics feature ongoingly in the institutions you belong to, knowledge of which is more often held in the breach. And it is within such a silence that a golem is made, and re-made. Together. The intergenerational transmission of trauma happens between as well as within persons, in intersubjective as well as social and historical space. We are haunted as much by what is not said as by what is done.

My experience of telling this story in its various iterations bears a bit of the uncanny too. When I tried to present it a second time, for example, I was nearly disinvited: What specter could have led a conference committee to declare that, as a patient recounting a transgression, I was in ethical breach because my (deceased) analyst—whom I have never publicly named—could not defend himself on grounds of having to keep confidentiality? What specter could have then caused a prominent psychoanalytic journal to "lose" a game-changing paper (Dimen, 2011) that both recounted the story of the transgression and analyzed the situation of sexual boundary violation in psychoanalysis? What specter could have even later brought down a conference planned to honor that very paper? Or turned a collection of papers dedicated to discussion of that selfsame paper into an anthology about the problem as a whole? What specter could subsequently cause another committee to acknowledge receipt of a new paper on the entire topic and then never announce they'd turned me down? Was it the same specter that, the next year, succeeded in disinviting the author of these works—me—from a keynote address?

Public 2

And yet. I must say that when it comes to the social dimensions of this weirdness, the ghost metaphor no longer cuts much ice. Begged are questions of personal and collective responsibility; one's relation toward these who are called here "ghosts;" gender; and power. Here we are in an area of much uncertainty for analysts.

The ghost made me, him, them do it? I don't think so. Writing of the false memory "syndrome" used to discredit those who have recovered memories of sexual abuse, Adrienne Harris (1996) says: "The demands made on the analyst to think, feel, reason, and process within a social field (the transference and countertransference phenomena) are anchored on a determination not to act but to reflect" (184).

Perhaps. But the distinction between action and reflection does not always hold. When it comes to actions, and patterns of action, and institutions that harm repeatedly, one wants to know how this nasty stuff happens, and how people come to it, and how one hurts another and how one enters into hurt. How does one enter the taboo, breaking laws willy-nilly? How does one opt for silence and erasure? How do groups do it? How do those who listen opt to do so? What are the vectors of power and pleasure in which our private and social beings take shape? How do these contingencies of desire pinball each of us into the infliction and reception of pain?

More. When these questions are asked by not one but many, is reflection no longer an action? When we agree to listen collectively, or just happen to do so, are we not also engaging an act? I do not know how to think this through alone. If you think it through with me, are we not also acting? Here goes.

Let me say it straightforwardly, even though to begin a paragraph this way is to be somewhat indirect: Colleagues hurt me, but—is this worse?—they may not have even registered how. And it embarrasses me to note these facts: in acknowledging the hurt, I am showing you something I'd rather you not see. Sometimes to acknowledge hurt risks seeming one-down, even sometimes a sense of abjection.

Still, if there is any purchase in the idea that the past lingers, then I am honor-bound to take that risk. "Why did you do that?" This is what I want to ask each of those who injured me in some way around this dilemma. My question is as much accusation as inquiry. Obscurely, though, I feel I am not supposed to accuse. I am only to think, reflect, consider, ponder, contemplate. And so I feel the impulse to drain the affect from these words, separate remonstration and indignation from reasoned inquiry into history and dynamics.

But perhaps separating the personal from the political, or the professional, is a stupid move. The ghosts of personal life meet the historical forces of public life, and they power each other. They animate the transgression, its excitement and guilt and pain. They vivify the objection, the protest, the outrage. As fascinated as one is by the haunting hurt and its *jouissance*, one still wants to, and must, say, even in the face of the unconscious: No.

Of course, I must blame each of the individuals who had some hand in these disappointing and sometimes shocking erasures. And yet so many smart and even compassionate people have acted like fools, as well as foolishly—and here I include Dr. O, and me too—that anyone with a sense of historical and cultural and psychological context must wonder what patterns are being relived despite our intent. Are these patterns historical? Social? Personal? All of the above, I think.

A "specter is haunting Europe." So wrote Karl Marx and Friedrich Engels about what they saw as a good thing, the communism that would create social justice and that society feared in the nineteenth century. But likening the ghosts of sexual boundary violations to "the specter of communism" doesn't quite work. After all, *The Communist Manifesto* is a work of irony, anger, passion: The "specter" Marx and Engels fingered was, in their view, desirable.

Can one write and speak with irony about sexual transgression? What would the equivalent specter be? Incest, of course, brims with desire. The wish for it, ever unresolved, spooks us at the oddest moments. It endures because the craving for the ecstasy that halos the violation of this universal taboo never abates (my own personal participation in which was stolen by Dr. O). Yet, speaking in the name of the law, decency, and what one is forced to call "mental health," incest stands outside the category of the desirable.

We face this problem with helplessness, irony beyond our shared reach, except of course in the gallows humor of the injured, in the jokes that cannot be told in front of them. Maybe it's better to think here of enigmas rather than golems, ghosts, specters, the uncanny. Perhaps we face an enigma: A specter is haunting psychoanalysis, the specter of enigma, enigma being inevitable and, perhaps, desirable in the work.

No. I don't think that works either.

"Don't mourn, organize!" This exhortation, attributed to the organizer Joe Hill executed for murder in 1915, capsules the problem.

Not that one either.

For psychoanalysis, can the ghost of sexual boundary violations become, one day, an ancestor (Loewald, 1960)? There is, of course, the problem that this sort of transgression is a contemporary, not a forebear: As I have been emphasizing, it inhabits the present as well as the past, and in all likelihood has a long, if maybe less robust future ahead. Many quote or render their own versions of Santayana's "Those who cannot remember the past are condemned to repeat it." In googling his aphorism, I ran into Kurt Vonnegut, who quips, "I've got news for Mr. Santayana: we're doomed to repeat the past no matter what. That's what it is to be alive" (http://www.goodreads.com/quotes/tag/doomed-to-repeat-it October 20, 2014).

Repetition does not exclude the new. Lives are hybrid, the past relived, the past corrected, the new created, the old uploaded, the seeds of the new secreted in the past. And suddenly one day, after decades and centuries of hard work, slavery is outlawed, women get the vote, health care becomes a public good, psychoanalysis joins the fray. That slavery endures elsewhere, that women remain disenfranchised somewhere else, that the public good is not as good as it should be and anyway is always under attack—that harm resurges—simply gives us more work to do.

What is the right way? Of litigation around sexual abuse, Harris (1996) has also written, "Whatever the many vicissitudes for a patient who has been abused and is attempting to come to terms with his or her experience, the goal of treatment in analysis is mourning a loss that cannot be undone with retribution nor perhaps even with justice" (166). Mourning, as opposed to melancholia, is classically thought to dispel the ghosts, but, as Judith Butler has argued (1995), Freud was wrong: Mourning is most always melancholia. Imbued with trauma, it is never really done, and so we survive in its penumbra of sadness, which serves as the somber grey sky against which the slanting sun looks ever more piercingly beautiful.

References

Butler, A. (1995). Melancholy—gender-refused identification. *Psychoanal. Dial.*, 5:165–180.
Dimen, M. (2011) "*Lapsus linguae*, or a slip of the tongue? A sexual violation in an analytic treatment and its personal and theoretical aftermath." *Contemp. Psychoanal.*, 47:36–79.
Falzeder, E. (2005–6). Psychoanalytic filiations. *Cabinet*, 20 http://www.cabinetmagazine.org/issues/20/falzeder.php, accessed December 22, 2014.
Harris, A. (1996), False memory? False memory syndrome? The so-called false memory syndrome? *Psychoanal. Dial.*, 6:155–187.
Herman, C. (2012). Sex with patient caused no harm, doctor says: Suit alleges negligence, violations of consumer law. *Commonwealth Magazine*, Winter 2012.
Loewald, H.W. (1960). On the therapeutic action of psycho-analysis. *Int. J. Psycho-Anal.*, 41:16–33.
Makari, G. (2008). *Revolution in Mind*. New York, NY: Harper Perennial.

Chapter 8

Basic uncertainty and totalitarian objects

Michael Šebek

"I do not know what to say . . . ", a young woman begins her session. Such a start is known to analysts as an introductory ritual, or simply repeating state of mind: a few seconds of uncertainty, something perhaps very fundamental, when the Ego is disoriented, not yet finding any content (object), state of confusion or chaos, a place for "ghosts" waiting for a free gate to consciousness, uncanny state of mind. She adds after a while: " . . . as it would not be me here!" showing feelings of strangeness and depersonalization, which are often a part of the whole picture and which indicate the presence of the uncanny. This introductory period, in which no representation is present, is sometimes so short that it is condensed in flashing silence although often it takes seconds or even minutes. Mostly patients finally find some words to express their unconscious fantasies, which is the classical domain of psychoanalysis seeking hidden meanings.

The same young woman after several sessions reflects on her initial uncertainty and uncanny feelings: " . . . connected with it, somehow . . . I feel also an urgent need of help, being strongly dependent on someone, on you, somebody strong who could keep me, save me, rather as if you would have a total power over my existence." This urgent need of the object in this basic conscious uncertainty seems to be more about survival than a libidinal cathexis; some would say "breast", or a primary object, but I prefer to use the term *saving object* to describe what I used to feel in such situations in my countertransference. Verbal expressions like "saving", "total power", "strongly dependent" are close to what I have defined some years ago as the *totalitarian object* (Šebek, 1996, 1998, 2000, 2001, 2012).

Another patient, more disturbed than the young woman mentioned above, starts his session with a desperate fall into uncertainty and emptiness: "Nothing to say . . . it is only chaos . . . ". After a while he feels "terrible rage", and adds: "as you are a tyrant, I am afraid of you . . . but I know you did not do anything wrong to me but you could . . . but I feel also strong dependence on you . . . like in prison, a paralysis . . . " Again a classical stage of psychoanalysis follows in his next sessions, when he discovers his mother functioning as "the tyrant" who actively took part in the communist repressions—but I want to follow moments of initial uncertainty and emptiness originating somewhere on the border between preconsciousness and consciousness, a temporal transitional space that is potentially creative, or a break that is felt as a blackout of the overwhelmed Ego, one of those unrepresented states which are today so much studied (see f.e. Botella & Botella, 2005; Levine, Reed & Scarfone, 2013;), and which are connected also with the study of the negative (Green, 2002). Logically these studies refer to Freud's fundamental work on the uncanny, negation, and the unconsciousness (Freud, 1915, 1919, 1925,). The feeling of uncertainty is a relative of the uncanny which so attracted Freud (Freud, 1919). The German word "*unheimlich*" can have various meanings but is associated with something strange, strangeness, something surprising, not expected, nor yet assimilated or even bizarre (de M'Uzan, 2009, 2013). Freud explained the uncanny as a return of the repressed and also archaic magic parts of psyche, which are still present today (Freud, 1912, 1919). Briefly, unconscious archaic objects operate in the uncanny, and may cause initial uncertainty and emptiness as a defense. This temporal space between unconscious presentations and conscious representations is a critical point in which, I believe, a *survival pattern* (*genetic programme* suggested by Michel de M'Uzan, 2013) is active, and a strong urge to attach to the external powerful and saving object is triggered. I have noticed many times in my clinical work that archaic saving objects (God-like omnipotent figures) or dangerous monsters, when traumatic moments prevailed in the past of a patient, are present in the transition between "nothing" (emptiness) and first representations. Fenichel (1940) described the dualistic character of Gods and God-like figures: goodness and badness. To save and to kill are much closer on the level of primary process. These archaic powerful objects may appear in a dream, in a fantasy (dream-like content), or in some nonverbal behavior and action f.e. the young women mentioned above, when on the sofa was suddenly flooded by a picture of a powerful monster—she quickly sat up to "escape" by acquiring more perceptual control in external reality (to see I am there behind her, and there is no monster).

I argue, that among primitive archaic objects with magic character, *the totalitarian object* has a special position, fulfilling at the beginning a saving function but through projection or projective identification, and also a direct experience with its materialized existence, it owns or acquires also persecutory and destructive drive elements. To illustrate this phenomenon I use the dream of the young woman whose introductory negation is described at the beginning:

> P: *What to say, what to catch, how to hold myself here, no content . . . (two minutes silence). Dreams always help, I am not responsible for them, but strange dreams! Only impression—nothing positive, but this I have said as an apology that it is not positive. Again it is about water, a river. I remember I am with my mum on the embankment, and I need to wash myself, I am jumping into the river, and the water becomes a bit wild with a lot of mud, I want to get out, it is the river somewhere in the forest. It is difficult to convey it, suddenly I am among many people, a mass, they are also swimming to the other embankment. It is a contest. Then I and others, many, are running through some town, but I cannot run so quickly, so all others are finally at the end, and I am a last one and I go to tell to organizers. Then I run a half of the whole distance back but I am running alone, I did not know that the contest is not going on back. So I am becoming disoriented, I do not remember the way, I am straying (blundering). Then I am in a hotel and besides me my client—girl—is in the bed. She is saying something humiliating for me, so I want escape but then some chap is joining us, and I pretend some politeness, but then I recognize in this man a hero-man from Hitchcock's Psycho. But I go somehow further and I am in a train. There is a mentally disturbed girl and I am expected to take care of her. But she keeps a normal conversation with a train conductor, and it would be impossible for me to do, and there is also a boy who was already present in the contest in the river and town. This boy has a tyre around his neck and wants to jump to a scarp. I have in my hand his letter saying goodbye. He starts to fall down, he starts to brake but it is not helping . . . chaos, pain, a fall from a rock, the net for suicides does not catch him . . . endless scene."*

I do not want to go into details of this rich dream but I want to focus on some parts, which are important for this study. When she had finished her dream story I felt paralyzed, I did not know "what to say", and it was uncanny.

I was her silent helpless "double"—the only difference was she was silent before the dream story, and I was after it. But "dream helps" she said—and she was right. We both could recover step by step from shadows of objects, which can be called "ghosts"(obviously ghosts behave like coming from some other ethereal world where we have no power and no reason, no words). Her "dream helps" means, that her Ego is already—after opening emptiness—oriented in the readable transference direction but some depersonalization (or a double) is also present: she does not feel "responsibility" for her dream content (not-me elements). The content is full of her mafia-persecuting totalitarian objects not allowing her any success, any progress, only a step-by-step devastating fall into a chasm. In this way her self or a series of her partial identities are owned and totally controlled by these totalitarian objects, sitting mostly in her superego and being projected in the transference on me (should the whole analysis fall down into a chasm?). The dream is not only uncanny, it is catastrophic, with a "Hitchcock's Psycho" ghost (one part of her hidden identity and the analyst in the transference). It is only several months later that the young woman can say about this dream (and several other very similar like this one): " . . . it is all me, Kafka's Process, my mafia is trying to kill me, my parents had a catastrophic relationship and my mum said to me when I was small that it was all (mother's catastrophic despair) caused by my birth, my existence!". So this kid should die in the oedipal triangle. It was Herbert Rosenfeld (1987) who indicated "mafia objects" disposing of a double function: protection and persecution. If this young woman were to "win" in her parental triangle (if she were to win in her contest in the dream content) it would be another catastrophe. Mafia objects are a specific type of what I call the *totalitarian object.*

In order to understand this concept and related processes better I need first to mention the work of Erik Erikson (1968) who suggested that the ego's synthetic function produces two qualitatively different "gestalts"/ syntheses. One is *totality*, and the other is *wholeness*. Wholeness, and alternatively *wholeheartedness, wholemindedness*, wholesomeness is an expression for healthy and organic interrelatedness of various functions and parts within entirety (mind) having at the same time open and fluid borders with the outside environment. Obviously, what Erikson means, is the functional and structural interrelatedness between ego, superego (ego-ideal involved), id, and the open and flexible borders with the outside environment. To add the object relation perspective to this: the inner objects are transformed into personal ideologies (Baranger & Baranger, 2009), perceptions and interpretation of the external objects in a way that corresponds more to reality than to reality distortion. This abstract description fits well with the concept of a normal adult personality not being based on the statistics but on multi-level functional confluences. Erikson then defines the totality as another way by which the entirety or gestalt is reached. The word "eclusive" was used by Erikson in the sense of of the senselusive" was used by Erikson in the sensehich the entirety or gestalt is reached.. and parts. There is an artificial delineation of what must remain outside, and what must remain inside—regardless of the logic of similarity and relatedness of events, processes and objects. Obviously the difference between good objects and bad objects is based on artificial (not based on normal experience) borders where nothing "between" is allowed and experienced. If an analyst becomes in the psychic reality of the patient a "devil" or Hitchcock's murderer, there is no space for anything good; alternatively, if he is represented as an idealized saviour, no fault is attributed to him. The same is true of ideologies connected with this split in the Ego. In the totalitarian mind there is no other possibility of additional choice or change. Ego closes itself in the black and white logic and personal ideologies have fixed rigid content and shape. Shortly there is no dialogue or discussion but only a monologue defining a closed space of totalitarian psyche.

We can see that the idea of totality goes beyond the clinical phenomena and enters the field of the complex adaptation of the mental apparatus to internal, as well as external, social reality. Returning to micro-processes, when the Ego starts to work in the initial "nothingness" (no content, no object, no representation) the initial transition (from unrepresented states, initial "no content", to archaic objects) can be done (not necessarily) by the primitive ego's synthetic function creating totality as the specific psychic organization.

Erikson's work on totality and wholeness remains practically unknown, and I think it needs some more elaboration.

In 1996 I wrote an article on **totalitarian objects**, and later elaborated on this topic (Šebek, 1996, 1998, 2000, 2001). The main characteristic of these originally archaic objects is their penetrating (aggressive), possessive, haunting and controlling function over the internal psychic space, and in this sense they are similar to mafia objects described by Herbert Rosenfeld. Totalitarian objects block the separation—individuation process, inhibit or destroy development to maturity (Erikson's wholeness), and help to create dogmatic ideologies (in which truth was already discovered!) in which creative thinking is not possible. When a person perceives the world through the lens of totalitarian objects seated mostly in the unconscious Ego, he/she conceives external objects as if they were in his or her possession, so that manipulation with them is possible. Totalitarian objects can find their place also in the split off-destructive self (Rosenfeld, 1971, 1987) or in the superego (severe, sadistic superego). They are also projected and the paranoid world starts to work. Totalitarian objects in their various forms can cause a negative therapeutic reaction or therapeutic impasse. Their almighty, omnipotent and omniscient character often allows an extreme and primitive idealization. Otto Fenichel (1940, 33–34) wrote about these archaic objects and connected them with uncanny feelings: "Now it is a strange thing with the Gods. The religion of all people and all times works with the fear which comes from the "uncanny"." He thinks that in the image of God itself, or in the cult, are many "archaic" features, which appear to bring back that which is old and overcome, in order to fill the believers with fear or awe and so keep a hold on them. The Gods have always had not only supernatural, but also underground, animal, and instinctual traits which one must fear. Furthermore, it is dangerous to have the sight of God, and many Gods of primitive races are very ugly. Fenichel wrote that totem animals and totemism were ancestors of religions, and many religious systems have a dualistic character: good and evil. "The devil is always more uncanny than God, always has more archaic characters, namely animal qualities, goats feet, horns, tail and ugliness" (35). I also believe *totalitarian objects* have in their archaic historical form and also in their new editions a dualistic nature: they cause uncanny feelings and fear, and at the same time they attract and fascinate (f.e. Stalin, Hitler). I suppose that the creation and the existence of these powerful objects fills the archaic gap between individual flimsy existence and the unpredictable dangerous forces in nature and culture (see Freud in The Future of an Illusion (1927) about human helplessness in the world of powerful forces as the root of religion). Puget (1992) proposed that besides the intrapsychic and interpsychic space there is the trans-subjective area involving the space between the individual and society. I think it is useful to involve in this area also nature, the cosmos, the endless space in which we are immersed since the birth, which is unconsciously the most undifferentiated part of oneself. This area is also not much symbolically expressed, and makes us feel ambiguous and chronically uncertain about the safety of the big world around us (see Sas, 2004, 2010). In our tendency to find out in any environment something familiar and safe (for the baby it is his mother as the resource of the basic trust, and for an adult it is any environment or people with whom he is familiar) we are specifically inclined to choose powerful objects which are endowed (in our perception and fantasy) with the capacity to meet our existential, trans-subjective distress, anxiety: they have saving (the idealized part) as well as persecuting (towards enemies) character. Inevitably both drives, libido and aggression, operate in these objects, and the *genetic programme*, too (see Michel de M'Uzan, 2013, who thinks that survival is not a "drive" but a "genetic programme"). But this power gives them the capacity of misuse, abuse and perverse solutions, and destructiveness may become their main characteristic. I believe that this trans-subjective area—being responsible in cultural macro-processes for the creation of Gods, religions and political ideologies—is ever present in psychic micro-processes, those I have described as initial uncertainty, initial strangeness, uncanny feelings and transitional depersonalizations at the beginning of psychoanalytic sessions (although they may occur at any time in the session), and probably also in ordinary life situations when the original mental setting involving habitual drive channels cannot be used in a new situation. For instance, people talk about uncanny feelings before and in new situations, or before meeting some important (powerful) people, before travelling to some new place, and a new (not yet known) adjustment is expected but not yet realized. In these uncertain situations drives must be newly redistributed and new "channels" to new objects need to be set up (see also de M'Uzan, 2013). Erikson thought that total psychic Ego solutions emerge in periods of transition from one developmental period to the next one. Obviously in these situations the Ego is not full master of the house, but is regressed, split or cannot yet find strategies for mastering new perceptions and redistribution of drives. At the beginning of a psychoanalytic session some transition from pre-session time and session time takes place and therefore the force of the unconscious is more felt: unconscious drives connected with primitive objects, "ghosts" and repressed conflicts/traumas push the psychic system into the trans-subjective area for a while, for seconds, sometimes for much longer. As a form of first progressive adjustment the totalitarian psychic organization with predominance of totalitarian objects may take the place: seeking a saviour or flight from a persecutory monster. All this can be traced a bit schematically as a chain:

(1) drive (psychic energy)—not yet directed to an object and causing uncertainty in the Ego;
(2) emergence of archaic objects;
(3) the ego total organization involving fixed beliefs and rigid patterns;
(4) the more differentiated object representations and the flexible ego organization based on wholeness.

The regressive steps back to basic uncertainty and (temporary) lack of representations are part of normal life.

Finally I want make some remarks of the usefulness of the concept of the totalitarian object and the Ego total synthesis. Erikson (1968) formed his theory in order to explain two things:

(1) mental states (developmental crisis) accompanying transitions between developmental stages;
(2) the attachment of masses of people to totalitarian regimes (particularly in Nazi Germany). He was convinced that external and internal totality must correspond to each other in some non-pathological way, too.

My view of the totalitarian object is based on similar but extended assumptions:

(1) Totalitarian régimes and tyrants existed repeatedly in human history, and they had to be maintained by people (see Plato in *The Republic*).
(2) Totalitarian objects are a silent part of culture. They existed before National Socialism and Communism and they are all the time the archaic part of the psyche—connected with survival needs in the trans-subjective space—helping to establish and maintain external totalitarian systems: totemism, Gods, religions, magic creatures, tyrants, dictators, various political and non-political ideologies and political extreme movements. Totalitarian objects can be internal and external and very often work together, though this is rarely recognized.
(3) External totalitarian figures (dictators, authoritarian leaders) and systems are easily uncovered by conscious perception but their internal counterparts remain unconscious and are even transmitted non—consciously from one generation to another.
(4) In this unrecognized "non-present" and unconscious form they function as ghosts, "present absences" (nothing), timeless objects of the unconscious

entering into a dream, behavior and conscious mental space—forming a specific transference and countertransference in psychoanalysis.
(5) In their historical and archaic form, totalitarian objects represent specific powerful ghosts of the past, parts of magic psyche described by Freud in Totem and Taboo (1912) and rediscovered in The Uncanny (1919).
(6) Totalitarianism of the twentieth century was originally planned as a saving system for the population traumatized by World War I and the economic crisis but it became the most destructive and uncontrollable force human mankind ever experienced. Therefore demonic forces, some sort of psychic malignity in human mind, exist. One way for the study of totalitarian objects is their connection with violence and trauma.
(7) Main transmitters of culture are parents. Many patients view their parents as totalitarian. They are described also as narcissistic and not empathic.
(8) Patients usually perceive their analysts as powerful authorities. Therefore the analytical process should avoid any coercion (Hinshelwood, 1997).
(9) An analyst in his countertransference may feel the temptation to govern, teach, direct and manipulate a patient—to be a saviour and idealized authority, or to be a persecutor and tyrant (in the patient's projection or without it). A patient who has "dictator" in his Ego wants to manipulate and direct his therapy and gives the analyst little chance to do any analytical work.

In our analytical patients we often observe that totalitarian objects are "incorporated" and hidden in rigid *beliefs* being a part of the total Ego synthesis. These *beliefs* are not necessarily only political, but more often represent guidelines for certain behaviors. They often play an important part in the safety of the self but they are obviously pathogenic (see also Sampson, 1994; Weiss, 1998), and may contain ghosts. For instance, the young woman whom I used to illustrate initial uncanny feelings believed that "to cry does not help anything and it is shame", in short, it is forbidden. The "author" (or one of authors) of this rigid belief was her father with whom she unconsciously identified. She could cry in analytic sessions relatively freely only after several years of analysis when some steps in her *wholeness* were already reached. Beyond this rigid belief the patient could discover a piece of the family history: a fortnight before her parents' wedding, her father's sister died in a mysterious bus accident. The wedding and funeral (mourning) were not ever integrated in the family, the death of sister was denied (the parents never talked about it with the patient) and the father's "crying does not help anything" had become a command for her emotional life. This ghost (dead aunt), Hitchcock's murder, Kafka's Process (she feels to be killed at the end), and "this kid caused a catastrophe and must die" in parental triangle, and finally the chronic circular negotiation with "mafia objects" (her parental figures)—all represent deeply interrelated patterns, ghostly and total, involving "no content" at the beginning of her sessions: " I do not know what to say . . . ."

Bibliography

Amati Sas, S. (2004). La interpretación en el trans-subjetivo; reflexiones sobre la ambigüedad y los espacios psíquicos. Revista de Psicoanálisis 57, 1, 129–139, Bs. As.; L'interprétation dans le trans-subjectif: réflexions sur l'ambiguïté et les espaces psychiques. Psychothérapie 24, 207–213, Genève; An interpretation in the trans-subjective space: some reflections on ambiguity and psychic space, EATGA - AETAG Newsletter, n.1, 2005.

Amati Sas, S. (2010). La transubjectivité entre cadre et ambiguïté. In Pichon M., Vermorel H., Kaës R. (a cura di), *L'expérience du groupe. Approche de l'œuvre de René Kaës*. 115–127. Paris: Dunod.

Baranger, M. & Baranger, W. (2009). *The Work of Confluence: Listening and Interpreting in the Psychoanalytic Field*. London: Karnac Books.

Botella, C. & Botella, S. (2005). *The Work of Psychic Figurability*. Hove: Brunner-Routledge.

Erikson, E.H. (1968). *Identity, Youth and Crisis*. London: Faber and Faber.

Fenichel, O. (1940): Psychoanalysis of antisemitism. *American Imago*, 1B: 24–39.

Freud, S. (1912). Totem and taboo. S.E. XIII.

Freud, S. (1915). The unconscious. S.E. XIV.

Freud, S. (1919). The uncanny. S.E. XVII.

Freud, S. (1925). Negation. S.E. XIX.

Freud, S. (1927). The future of an illusion. S.E. XXI.

Green, A. (2002). *The Work of the Negative*. London: Free Association Books.

Hinshelwood, R.D. (1997). *Therapy or Coercion: Does Psychoanalysis Differ From Brainwashing?* London: Karnac Books.

Levine, H.B., Reed, G.S. & Scarfone, D. (2013). *Unrepresented States and the Construction of Meaning*, London: Karnac Books.

de M 'Uzan, M. (2013). *Death and Identity*. London: Karnac Books.

de M 'Uzan, M. (2009). The uncanny or "I am not who you think I am". Chapter 9 in M. de M 'Uzan, *Death and Identity* (2013). London: Karnac Books.

Puget, J. (1992): Belonging and ethics. *Psychoanal. Inq.*, 12, 551–569.

Rosenfeld, H. (1971). A clinical approach to the psychoanalytic theory of the life and death instincts. An investigation into the aggressive aspects of narcissism. *Int. J. Psychoanal.* 52, 169–178.

Rosenfeld, H. (1987). *Impasse and Interpretation*. London: Tavistock.

Sampson, H. (1994). Repeating pathological relationships to disconfirm pathogenic beliefs: Commentary on Steven Stern's "Needed relationship". *Psychoanal. Dial.* 4, 357–361.
Šebek, M. (1994). The true self and the false self: The clinical and social perspective. *J. British Assoc. of Psychotherapists.* 26, 22–39.
Šebek, M. (1996). The fate of the totalitarian object. *Intern. Forum of Psychoanalysis,* 5, (4) 289–24.
Šebek, M. (1998). Post-totalitarian personality – old internal objects in a new situation. *J. Am. Academy Psychoanal.,* 26 (2), 295–309.
Šebek, M. (2000). Das Schicksal der totalitaren Objekte. Wo stehen wir mit unseren Patienten? In: Kerz-Ruhling, I. et al. (Hrsg.): *Sozialistische Diktatur und psychische Folgen.* Tubingen: Sigmund-Freud-Institut, Psychoanalytische Beiträge 4. pp. 197–216.
Šebek, M. (2001). Zeit, Raum und Gedachtnis fur totalitare Objekte, In: Werner Bohleber and Sibylle Drews (Eds.), *DieGegenwart der Psychoanalyse – die Psychoanalyse der Gegenwart.*, Stuttgart: Klett-Cotta.
Šebek, M. (2012). Destins des objets totalitaires. In: H. Vermorel, G. Carbol and H. Parat (Eds.). *Guerres Mondiales Totalitarismes, Genocides.* Paris: EDK.
Weiss, J. (1998): Patient's unconscious plans for solving their problems. *Psychoanal. Dial.,* 8, 411–428.

Chapter 9

The presence of the past
Transmission of slavery's traumas

Janice P. Gump

I am grateful to the editors of *Demons in the Consulting Room* for selecting slavery within which to examine the intergenerational transmission of trauma. One might exclaim "But of course!" as this was the most visible, societally determining trauma this country has ever known, and the source of the most devastating war to take place on our soil. And yet, though a frequent topic in history and the social sciences, the trauma of slavery has been little considered from a psychological or psychoanalytic perspective.

Political as well as economic and cultural factors have played a role in this silence. In *Inhuman Bondage: The Rise and Fall of Slavery in the New World*, David Brion Davis (2006) writes that at the end of the Civil War there were two "seemingly contradictory but widely held views of the War's significance" (p. 304). Former president Jefferson Davis maintained "'slavery was in no wise the cause of the conflict, but only an incident.'" But, Davis (2006) notes, there were also those who held slavery's abolition to be the greatest "crime of the 19th century . . . (in which case) slavery must have been something more than 'an incident'" (p. 304).

Davis (2006) describes a plethora of novels and memoirs published from the 1800s through 1950 "extolling the agrarian utopia of the South in which devoted "mammies" and other loyal slaves not only exemplified racial harmony but dramatized a relationship between worker and "employer" that transcended all conflict . . . "

As a descendant of slaves, the above astounds me. Given the act of African enslavement, the Middle Passage during which almost 2 million Africans died (Gates, 2014), rape, psychological as well as physical abuse, captivity enforced by laws, fences, and roaming "pattyrollers" who beat slaves found outside plantation boundaries, the selling of mothers from children, fathers from families, siblings divided and separately sold, the prohibition of learning, and finally, the all-encompassing, irremediable message of "defective", the contention of slavery's benevolence is stunning. Only if slaves were governed by laws other than those regarding humanity as a whole could the thesis be found acceptable. Such beliefs, however, as well as the denial undergirding them, continue to haunt both descendants and the nation.

The descendants and following quote conveys what I contend. From 1936–1938 the Federal Writers' Project had interviewers record the narratives of ex-slaves. One compilation of the more than 2,000 collected was published by Yetman (2002). The following passage is taken from that source. The narrator is 100-year old Delia Garlic:

> I was born at Powhatan, Virginia, and was the youngest of thirteen chillen. I never seed none of my brothers and sisters 'cept brother William. Him and my mother and me was brought in a speculator's drove to Richmond and put in a warehouse with a drove of other niggers. Den we was all put on a block and sold to de highest bidder. I never seed brother William again.
>
> Mammy and me was sold... (to) de sheriff of de county... He was a widower and his daughter kept house for him. I nursed for her and one day I was playin' with de baby. It hurt its li'l hand and commenced to cry and she whirl on me, pick up a hot iron and run it all down my arm and hand. It took off de flesh when she done it.
>
> After a while, Marster married again, but things weren't no better. I seed his wife blackin' her eyebrows with smut one day, so I thought I'd black mine just for fun. I rubbed some smut on my eyebrows and forgot to rub it off, and she cotched me. She was powerful mad and yelled: 'You black devil, I'll show you how to mock your betters.' Den she pick up a stick of stovewood and flails it against my head. I didn't know nothin' more till I come to, lyin' on de floor. I heard de mistis say to one of the girls, 'I thought her thick skull and cap of wool could take it better than that.'

Delia continues to work on the plantation until one night, when she is serving her drunk master, "his head lollin'," he looks at her. She is frightened, which angers him, and he orders an overseer to:

'Take her out and beat some sense in her.' I begin to cry and run and run in de night, but finally I run back by de quarters and heard Mammy callin' me. I went in, and right away dey come for me. A horse was standin' in front of de house, and I was took dat very night to Richmond and sold to a speculator again. I never seed my mammy anymore.

(pp. 43–44)

I initially included this quote with the hope that as readers learned more about slavery they would also come to know the affects it produced. Though Delia articulates little of those affects, it is difficult *not* to imagine them. But this quote, like many of the narratives, reveals not just affects, but cognitive/affective/ relational *principles* of subjectivity. I experienced a hopeless helplessness in this woman, which, though it reflected the reality of her life, needs to be distinguished from that reality. It was not just that circumstances had rendered her helpless, but that that reality had become a principle of her subjectivity. It would determine how she would relate to others—a mate, Union troops, her own offspring—as well as determine a sense of agency, that is, a capacity to formulate goals, to plan their attainment and to be self-reflective in their actualization.

The consequences of traumas such as Delia suffered—an impoverished sense of self and resultant sense of impotence and agentic deficiency—became defining of who she was in the world, principles of her subjectivity. And such principles have been transmitted to descendants.

I shall use Atwood and Stolorow's (2014) understanding of trauma and relevant constructs in discussing several topics. Initially I will present their conceptualization of trauma. Subjectivity will then be examined, or rather, structures of subjectivity, which are "the distinctive configurations of self and other that shape and organize a person's subjective world" (p. 28). The slave's subjectivity is one manner in which the "what" of transmitted trauma may be determined, and I will discuss those aspects I find most significant, as well as give examples of its manifestation in present-day descendants. All of the patients I present are African American.

It is difficult to imagine descendants *not* haunted, in varying degrees, by the matters discussed. The traumas of slavery and their transmission are thus relevant to the therapy of all African Americans, whether made explicit or not. Therapists working with African American patients need have such knowledge. But the culture's treatment of African Americans is relevant not only to blacks, but to whites as well, because they too have been determined by it. It is this determination which Lynne Jacobs writes of in *Psychoanalytic Inquiry's Analytic Lives in a Wounded World* edition (2014, v.34). Both Jacobs' paper and my response to it (2014) discuss the work in which whites need engage in order for racism's effect upon *whites* to become clear. It is, after all, as necessary for the white therapist to know self as to know other, and this aspect of the self is particularly important in part because it is less visible.

I will also explore slavery's injurious impact upon the slave's sense of self, an impact which has been transmitted as well. My chapter will close with a discussion of transmission.

Trauma

The term "trauma" has been used to describe a wide array of psychological states, ranging from caregiver-infant interactions to the shattering and devastating effects of war, rape, and concentration camp phenomena. Atwood and Stolorow (2014) define the term in a manner that identifies the central phenomenon common to all.

For more than two decades these theorists and others (Stolorow & Atwood, 1992; Stolorow, Atwood & Brandchaft, 1994; Brandchaft, 1994; Orange, Atwood & Stolorow, 1997; Stolorow, Atwood & Orange, 2002) have maintained that trauma comprises an unbearably painful affective state which fails to be met with a containing, modulating, and regulating response. The relational context is essential to their thinking, indeed to their very definition of trauma. Trauma is not an external or even internal event, but the experiencing of unbearable affects in a *context* wherein modulating, containing, integrating responsivity fails to occur. It is this contextual process of which trauma is comprised.

The trauma of slavery

I have often used the word trauma to refer to events taking place during slavery. Though such use is appropriate, it is misleading, for it obscures the fact that the state of slavery in and of itself was traumatic. For instance, the most fundamental principle of slavery was the contention that blacks were inferior to whites, inadequate, and defective—in fact, not-quite-human. This belief preceded slavery, as it was born of European colonists' earliest encounters with black Africa (Frankenberg, 1993). We can see this principle concretized in the definition of slaves as "property", and the sale and purchase of them along with other properties. In the evaluation preceding the sale of goods, properties were ranked according to value: horses and men were equal in worth, as were cattle and women, and pigs and children. Such practices produced a reality which reinforced notions of inequality. Enforced detainment within the boundaries of the plantation, whether through the use of patrollers or locks placed on huts at night, was a kind of imprisonment, restricting information about the world, and one's self in relation to it.

And finally, it was the *state* of slavery that made possible the particular traumas occurring within it. For example, laws were established, such as the necessity of written permission to travel outside the plantation, the breaking of which permitted those who found such a slave to physically abuse him or her. Here we see a particular trauma, which owes its existence to the institution.

Developmental trauma

The work of Socarides and Stolorow (1984/1985) played a significant role in the conceptualization of affect as the primary motivator in human behavior, replacing drive which had, in psychoanalysis, been viewed as the primary motivator. That work also grasped the necessity of intersubjective experience in the integration of affects. Thinking in terms of the centrality of affect and its occurrence within ongoing relational systems made it possible for Atwood and Stolorow (2014) to rethink many psychological phenomena. Trauma was one of them.

When an infant or child experiences an intensely painful affective state within a context where pain is neither contained nor modulated, the affect becomes unbearable. It is the failure of the caretaker's *attunement* which renders these states unbearable, and which prevents their integration. Atwood and Stolorow (2014) hold that in such instances the child loses the capacity for integrating affect, and "unintegrated affect states become the source of lifelong emotional conflict and vulnerability to traumatic states because they are experienced as threats both to the person's established psychological organization and to the maintenance of vitally needed ties" (p.104). Such traumas have been labeled developmental trauma, a trauma many slaves endured. They are the most formative and enduring traumas, leading not only to the child's loss of affect-integrating capacity, but to the establishment of irremediable principles of organization which can be altered neither by conscious intent or later experience (Brandchaft, 1994).

Further, if these painful states have repeatedly evoked malattunement, the child comes to believe, unconsciously, that this malattunement and loss must derive from his own inherent defectiveness, his irreparable badness. This can be the source of lifelong and intense shame.

A patient I saw many years ago presented a powerful demonstration of such processes and results. The patient was chronically depressed, and felt acutely inadequate and guilty around her lack of desire for children. Clinically she was anxious and hysterical, and possessed an elusive kind of inappropriateness. She had "wack attacks" in which she would cry hysterically and hit her head against a wall, manifesting the overwhelmed, disorganized state Atwood and Stolorow (2014) cite as one outcome of malattunement.

Both she and her husband considered her immature and irresponsible about the mechanics of life (e.g., paying bills, meeting him at prearranged times). For years she took clothes to a laundromat because she couldn't decide whether to have the garbage disposal or the washing machine fixed first, or how to go about doing either. Genetic work was difficult, as the patient could not accept that parents as "wonderful" as hers could in any way bear responsibility for her confusion and misery. Indeed, her mother and father were the envy of her friends, as they were warm, open, and interested. Kids gathered at the patient's home as much to talk with her parents as with her. Both mother and father were well regarded professionally.

The father's birth and early childhood were mysterious. No one could (would?) ever tell my patient how he happened to be born on an Indian reservation. Though the family occasionally saw his mother, there was much distance between them. The father never spoke of his early history.

The father revered his wife, who was from a more privileged background, and adored his child. Theirs was the perfect home, there being no acknowledgement of father's rage which, subterranean, ruled the household through threats of eruption.

"That's why he had to have another family", the patient explained, for father's rage would have spoiled what he esteemed the most, his wife and my patient. And so, to protect them, and to keep from imploding, he created a receptacle in which his anger could be tolerated—a second, secret family. There he slept with a gun under his pillow. For the most part this father appeared to manage his rage through a dissociative process.

Father cared for the patient in infancy and early childhood, and it was he who taught her emotions. He would grimace and say, "Now what's this?" and the patient would respond "anger", or "what's this?" and she would say "surprise". Her recognition of feeling was to be from the outside in: it was not *her* anger, disappointment, or sadness which was to be labeled, for what could *she* know of such feeling? And should something slip through, father would say, "What's the matter with your face? Fix it". Affects were qualities to be acquired through careful instruction.

It was, she told me, a profound and critical point in our work when, angry at me, she leapt from her chair and began to walk. I quietly suggested she sit down, and experience what she was feeling. She told me it was the first time she had ever felt anger.

It need be remembered that my patient's principal early caregiver had been her father, a man whose history, personality, and relationship to his daughter suggest that in all probability he had experienced severe pain, which had failed to be modulated or contained. His presentation of self as kind and loving within my patient's family—certainly not the kind of man who would go to bed with a gun under his pillow—and his establishment of a secret second family, which my patient and mother learned of only when he died, suggest, as I've noted, dissociative characterology.

The father's history is highly suggestive, if not indicative, of trauma. What could have led to his birth and childhood on an Indian reservation, a context so different from that which most African Americans experienced? And what *had* been the nature of his relationship with his mother, whom he rarely saw, and whom his daughter found strange and difficult to relate to? Finally, the very nature of his daughter's care, one that held that feelings were not intrinsic, but had to be taught, and that some were impossible for *her* to have, strongly suggested the lack of integration of such painful affects within himself.

This case is a dramatic instance of developmental trauma: not only does an initial instance of a child's painful affect fail to be met with a modulating, containing response, but the caregiver makes clear that the enhanced pain resulting from the first malattunement will be punished. "You are allowed to feel joy, excitement, surprise: Sadness, anger, or disappointment is forbidden, and the consequence will be severe should you make a mistake". Father had made it abundantly clear he would not only be malattuned, but critical, and sometimes angry. It is the experience of pain *within such a context* that renders the child's state unbearable. And it is the repetition of such interactions that produces the "disorganized state".

Mother's role in these interactions seems to have been minimal, but in any case it is clear father's messages prevailed. What was transmitted, then, was what must have been father's experience of malattunement: when he was in pain, a response which contained and soothed failed to come forth. I have wondered if the father's mother was even present. But whether present or not, emotional holding appears absent, and her son thus lacked what was needed to hold his own child. Though many might speak of mother's ghost in such interactions, I prefer the word "haunted", which I discuss at greater length in the section on Transmission. My sense, however, is that though unable to modulate and contain his child's greatest pains, he had somehow still learned to give her much he never had.

When I worked with this patient I knew less about trauma and its transmission than I do today. I had less comprehension of an aloneness which must have been unbearable; I can't help but think I would have had greater empathy had I known. Nonetheless, the patient became more accepting of forbidden feelings, and both her disorganized state and depression diminished. She went back to school for an additional degree and her professional life matured.

The slave's subjectivity

Though my knowledge of slaves' subjectivity was enhanced by the slave narratives, it was Frederick Douglass' 1845 (Gates, 1987) autobiography, given its insight and eloquence, which heightened my historical and affective understanding. Gates captured my experience of Douglass' work when he wrote in the introduction, "Douglass's rhetorical power convinces us that he is 'the' black slave, that he embodies the structures of thoughts and feelings of all black slaves, that he is the resplendent, articulate part that stands for the whole . . . " (p. xiii).

Subjugation

The first principle of slavery was subjugation (Gump, 2010), for which Random House (1966, 1967) offers two definitions. "Bringing under complete control or subjection" is the first definition. The second is "to make submissive or subservient, to enslave". The dictionary thus distinguishes these related meanings, with the first relating to power or control, and the second to subservience or submission. The African was indisputably controlled by his master, made to work at whatever task for however many hours, allotted shelter, food and clothing according to the master's dictates, etc. But I glean from my reading most masters *also* demanded subservience: indeed, it appears that much of the violence towards slaves occurred in pursuit of this objective.

The term "broken" is frequently used in discussions of slavery. I came to understand that the process of "breaking" a slave referred to the success of subjugation. Frederick Douglass (Gates, 1987) eloquently describes this experience. Due to deaths in his master's family Douglass had had to leave the master's son with whom he first lived and come to live with another son, a "slaveholder destitute of every element of character commanding respect" (p. 286). This son does not like Douglass, and after nine months sends him to live with a poor "farm-renter", who was widely regarded for his ability to break slaves. Having never been a field hand, Douglass is awkward, and the first week of his stay he is given a task with unbroken oxen, with disastrous result. Mr. Covey beats him savagely, initiating a pattern that occurs almost weekly.

> If at any one time of my life more than another, I was made to drink the bitterest dregs of slavery, that time was during the first six months of my stay with Mr. Covey. We were worked in all weathers. It was never too hot or too cold; it could never rain, blow, hail, or snow, too hard for us to work in the field . . . The longest days were too short for him, and the shortest nights too long. I was somewhat unmanageable when I first went there, but a few months of this discipline tamed me. Mr. Covey succeeded in breaking me. I was broken in body, soul and spirit. My natural elasticity was crushed, my intellect languished, the disposition to read departed, the cheerful spark that lingered about my eye died; the dark night of slavery closed in upon me; and behold a man transformed into a brute!
> (Gates, 1987, p. 293)

Though having been severely beaten by Mr. Covey, Douglass determines to walk the seven miles to his master's store to ask that he be removed. His request is refused and he is returned. And then, one day, Covey intentionally surprises him, causing Douglass to fall. "But at this moment – from whence came the spirit I don't know – I resolved to fight". He does, and wins the immediate and larger battle:

> This battle was the turning-point in my career as a slave. It rekindled the few expiring embers of freedom, and revived within me a sense of my own manhood . . . and inspired me again . . . to be free . . . I now resolved that however long I might remain a slave in form, the day had passed forever when I could be a slave in fact."
>
> (Gates, 1987, pp. 298–299)

Though, as Gates (1987) wrote, Douglass spoke for all slaves, his courage, intelligence, and strong sense of self also reveal how unique he was, in spite of an early history seemingly profoundly lacking in what we regard as essential. His mother was taken from him upon his birth. He was told that in his infancy she had four times walked seven miles to be with him as he slept. He never saw her following those visits: she died when he was four. One has to wonder whether there wasn't *someone* who provided some degree of that psychological caretaking we regard as critical. But even had there been, would not there remain the yawning hole of the "real" mother, who has been snatched away, to be seen only rarely or never?

Slavery necessitated that children be cared for by others, sometimes to the degree that another's child be raised as one's own. I don't know Douglass' early life, but given what he became, and what I know of black culture, I strongly suspect there was someone.

A sense of self

Douglass' (Gates, 1987) ultimate sense of self in his struggles with the slave breaker are pronounced and triumphant, making the relevance of this construct incontrovertible in a consideration of slavery's effects. I suspected that though transitory, the sense of self was an authentic, perhaps even exultant experience in which one felt affirmed.

Brandchaft's (1994) sense of self construct confirmed my feelings. He describes a defensive process initiated when the child's efforts "to use his own feelings as central organizers of experience and behavior were stifled by attitudes and actions of caretakers" (p. 63). Describing his work with a patient who struggles to hold on to a sense of self he writes, "There is an underlying process at work . . . that discloses skeletons below. Within this skeletal framework experience is being shaped sequentially by two different and incompatible perspectives . . . " (p. 62).

One perspective is that of the child, who has the sense that his feelings can be used to organize his behavior and experiences. "(But) his own feelings (are) stifled by attitudes and actions of caretakers . . . Thus the perspective and motivation that prevails is one in which the individual is compelled to submit to a definition of himself determined by forces external to his control or volition, a definition determined by the needs, wishes and fears of caregivers or those who continue to represent them psychically" (p. 63).

Further, Brandchaft (1994) holds that "The most serious and lasting damage incurred by developmental traumata is that sustained by the emerging and fragile sense of self . . . (Though) each step toward the realization of a demarcated and authentic personality . . . is initially but fleetingly accompanied by a vitalizing and transcendent sense of self" (p 70), in instances where the sense of self is translocated it is followed by "the malaise and depletion of defeat and surrender . . . rooted in (an) underlying shift in the foundations of the sense of self" (p. 71).

My patient Marissa has struggled to achieve a sense of self. An intelligent, pretty, middle-aged woman, she presented with the issue of her husband, who was psychologically abusive, controlling, self-absorbed, and cruel. She had wanted to leave him for years, due to his physical abuse of their children and mismanagement of their funds, as well as his treatment of her. After three years of twice weekly therapy, and a period of couples work with another therapist, she engaged an attorney and obtained a divorce.

Marissa was soft spoken and mild mannered. Affect was largely absent, except for a muted quality of fearfulness—there was something ghostlike about her. She was afraid to challenge the desires of her husband, phobic about driving, employed for 12 years in a setting where she felt less-than and unappreciated.

Her flatness of affect was difficult for me to fathom. Even when, during the course of our work, a child with a chronic and serious illness died, the patient exhibited a constricted grief, not in keeping with her devotion and love for this child. The construct sense of self was instructive.

My patient was the daughter of upper-middle class African American parents who lived in a southern town. The father was a professional, the mother a school teacher. The mother made clear her preference for my patient's older sibling. A picture of the two children was revealing: the preferred child, dressed in a favorite outfit, smiling, is clearly the subject of the photograph. My patient, about two years old, is sitting on a curb a good distance away from her sibling, looking at her fingers, a look both sad and lost on her face. "Who is *that,*" one wonders, "and what is she doing in this picture!"

Marissa's mother reiterated her disappointment in her daughter often: she was too dark, her hair wasn't straight enough, her taste in clothes no good. It was blatantly clear she thought her less attractive than was she. Later, mother told her her friends were ugly, no boys would be interested in them and therefore in her. And mother's abuse was not all verbal, for she would slap and hit the patient, or have the father beat her.

Once my patient and brother took a trip with their mother to a city far removed from their home. They stayed in a hotel, and in leaving took an elevator to reach their car. My patient, age seven, pushed the wrong button in the elevator: mother began to scream: "You stupid idiot! Look what you've done! Now they'll think something is wrong, or that these ignorant black people are deliberately trying to cause trouble and they'll never let us stay here *again!* How could you be so dumb!" And she excoriated her, with the aid of the older sibling, for the entire seven-hour length of the trip, according to my patient. The episode wounded her so deeply, I doubt she is exaggerating.

Marissa's mother was the daughter of someone who had suffered considerable trauma. The grandmother as a child lived with her mother in the home of a family for whom the mother worked. The grandmother was the product of the master's rape of her mother. Many of slavery's customs, such as this one, survived its demise. When the grandmother was 12, her mother died, and the grandmother was sent away. I believe she married twice, initially to escape an insufferable situation, the second time to someone she loved, a physician. And then he died. She experienced poverty and the weight of raising three children on her own. She mothered her daughter much as her daughter mothered my patient, with anger and abuse.

A year after leaving her husband my patient obtained other employment, where she has exhibited increasing and appropriate assertiveness. Her subjugation has diminished significantly. In addition, she has bought her own home.

About a year ago we reached an impasse in the treatment. Though she had gained considerable independence, interacted with others in a manner both more protective and revealing of self, in the therapeutic work her intersubjective persona seemed untouched. She would ask my help with minutiae at work, she would tell me about self-help books she was reading—she gave us little to work on. I decided to seek consultation. And while she also felt we had reached an impasse, she had with reason become genuinely concerned about money. We dropped down to once a week, a temporary solution to the larger issues.

She had been reading Toni Morrison's *The Bluest Eye*, a novel replete with the trauma African American children experience from parents. We spoke of her mother's hostility towards her, of her grandmother's similar treatment of her mother, and I said something about how far back the absence of holding in our people goes: the trauma of initial capture, the long walk to the holding pens, the dankness and darkness of those pens as experienced by a contemporary African American journalist, the trauma of the ship's crossing where the vertical height of typical slave compartments was 18 inches, the deaths of almost 2 million Africans in those journeys, and what they encountered when they finally arrived... We were both open to the anguish of it, experiencing a simultaneity never before achieved. I had never been in such a place *with* anyone, and I am confident neither had she.

It is difficult to describe what happened. Near the end of my list of slave wounds I felt near tears for a moment, and as I looked at my patient realized she did as well. She shed a few, but I had moved past my sadness to the *incredulity* of the devastation wrought us (18" compartments?!) and she was again with me. It was as if we had experienced our sorrow, accepted it, and now, deeply informed, could be amazed at what had befallen us.

Clearly, the therapeutic impasse has to do with a maternal transference, one that remains to be worked through. In the moments described, however, our transferences fell and we met as equals who had suffered our mothers' voids, voids created by traumas of hundreds of years. It was *these* traumas, transmitted by mother that gave my patient a ghostlike quality: "How could you be so mean, mom? So indifferent to my feelings, so subjugating, so uncaring of your effect upon me?" Such thoughts were unconscious, but the affects they articulated were present and strong. And I am maintaining that it is the *affects* evoked by mother's acts, evoked ultimately by slavery's acts, acts not known to consciousness, which haunted her.

At the beginning of the hour above described, the patient had told me an anecdote in which someone she was working with had erred and was apologetic. My patient had said in a light, warm tone, "Oh! So you're human!" I had never heard her as empathic, as light, as charming. During the session I realized that until recently I had been responding to a deadened sense of self—that it was not just her affect that was flat, but that her whole being was deadened. The inflection, tone and smile accompanying "Oh! So you're human" was wonderfully alive.

The transmission of trauma is clear in this instance. The grandmother's mother had endured trauma in the house where she lived, and undoubtedly the traumas of earlier generations had been transmitted to her as well. She then transmitted traumas to her child, the grandmother, amongst them her death, who in turn transmitted traumas to my patient's mother, who conveyed them to her daughter, my patient. There is a void in these women where there needed to be a capacity to react in a containing, holding manner, a void the original source of which was slavery. This is my understanding of the Dead Mother phenomenon, which I discuss below at greater length.

In what follows I shall explore two components of the sense of self, agency, and the proscription of affect.

Agency

Destruction of the slave's agency was critical to slavers and critically impairing of the slave. Bandura (2001) broadly defines agency as "the capacity to exercise control over the nature and quality of one's life" (p. 1). He is referring to a capacity to desire, to formulate goals, to make relevant plans, to evaluate one's ability to enact such plans and then bring them about, in short, to have purpose, direction, and meaningfulness in one's life. With, I would add, a resultant sense of potency.

For the most part, agentic faculties were antithetical to the institution of slavery, and not only were slaves held incapable of performing them, slave narratives suggest that in fact slaves were deficient in this regard. The following quote from ex-slave Anthony Dawson's narrative (Yetman, 2002) describes such a deficiency.

> The niggers kept talking about being free about being free, but they wasn't free then and they ain't now. ('Now' is 1936 or '37). Putting them free just like putting goat hair on a sheep. When it rain de goat come a-running and get in de shelter 'cause his hair won't shed the rain and he get cold, but de sheep ain't got sense enough to get in the shelter but just stand out and let it rain on him all day. But the good

Lord fix the sheep up with a woolly jacket that turn the water off, and he don't get cold, so he don't have to have no brains. De master's protection was like de woolly coat. But de 'mancipation come and take off de woolly coat and leave de nigger with no protection and he cain't take care of hisself either. (p.29)

Most statements of being adrift were not as creative, but spoke to the reality of the freed slave's situation: he was without money, knew little or nothing of what lay outside the plantation, and had no immediate job possibilities except those the master might offer. And so most of the ex-slaves' families in Yetman's (2002) collection remained on their plantations, now working for minimal sums.

It is clear that what was *done* to slaves produced the deficiencies of function they were then demeaned for lacking. How could someone held captive, forced to perform according to another's demands, controlled in almost every aspect of their existence possess agency?

The proscription of affects and desire

Slavery demanded the slave's surrender of a sense of self. He must give up wanting—shoes, his wife's continued presence, self-determined goals. I had believed this for many years, but it was a recent memory of me with my father that helped me understand the proscription of desire within black families. I no longer remember why my father was in a position where, from time to time, he would have boxes of candy. Perhaps he was connected in some way to wholesale goods, but for whatever reason on occasion boxes of candy bars were stored in our hall closet. One day I decided to take one, and he caught me. "***What*** are you ***doing!***?" he said loudly and with incredulity. I muttered that I wanted one. "Who ***cares*** if you ***want*** one" he responded with anger and mocking. I want a million dollars too. **So what?**"

I have written (2014) of my father, who, at the age of eight, was sent away from his family to live with a relative, and essentially raised himself. This very intelligent, poised, attractive man had struggled enormously to provide for us, as for most of his life he had been forced to accept occupations far beneath his capabilities, due to racism. He had periods of severe depression where he would sit motionless on the couch for hours, perhaps listening to Bach, responding only with a faint smile when I sought to engage him. I knew something was terribly wrong, and given the conversations I had overheard, surmised his state was due to all that he yearned for but seemed unable to acquire, despite immense effort. How selfish of me to think I should have what I wanted. I was not just guilty, but ashamed. Numerous iterations of such responses taught me to inhibit desire.

Slavery prohibited dysphoric affects, anger, and desire. Sadness rebuked the notion of slavery's goodness, and could interfere with functioning. It was foolishly dangerous to be angry, to show resentment for some affront or command. My father's personal history made his depressions understandable, but only recently did I realize I was witnessing trauma transmitted.

"Proscription", used in the heading of this section means, "to denounce or condemn ... as dangerous or harmful" (*Oxford English Dictionary* (1966). It could be dangerous for the slave to ask for what he wanted, such as three rather than two meals. And the child could be condemned—and certainly not cuddled—for asking for what she desired. Those slaves who were brought here, who were torn from all that was comforting and familiar, even to the point of being separated from those who spoke as they did—may have experienced attunement prior to capture, but would probably have little of it available given the traumas endured. How can a slave parent so treated, listen, accept the anger and tears, sometimes loud wails of a child's disappointment? And when their descendants ask parents for a two-wheel bicycle, a lack of empathy is not surprising. Who cares what you want?

The dead mother

Gerson (2009) explores the psychological impact of the Holocaust's traumas upon its survivors. A phenomenon witnessed clinically as well as socially in survivors and their children is one in which absence itself becomes the abiding presence. And it is an absence not just of the deceased mother, who had been the source of care and containment, but also of the *symbolic* representation of those functions she performed. Gerson cites the work of Andre Green, whose understanding of this "presence of a sense of absence at the core" led to the "poignant metaphor of the Dead Mother" (p. 6). This concept not only conveys the magnitude of anguish brought about by such loss, but speaks to the traumatic withdrawal of provision and care from a source previously relied upon, whose nurturance is expected in the future. There is now a void where once there had been not only a soothing warmth and containment, but the expectation of its repetition. Further, such trauma goes beyond literal loss and results in permanent damage to related internal structures. It is difficult *not* to think of attachment theory, and the significance Bowlby attached to internal working models as determiners of future behavior (Cassidy, 1999).

This emptiness, Gerson (2009) maintains, is now transmitted to the child. It is not clear how transmittal of this emptiness occurs, but through some unconscious process the survivor's child receives the blankness and deadness of the mother's traumatic loss, in place of the holding and providing care which the child requires. Further, the survivor comes to experience the world as unresponsive to her suffering, and uncaring of her fate, which was the way many Holocaust survivors and their descendants felt.

I am seeing a patient whose history is extraordinary with regard to a mother's inability to hold. As a child, my patient suffered the inevitable childhood cuts and abrasions. Her mother would respond with indifference or irritation to such wounds, as in "Get up off that floor and *stop* that crying!" without examining the source of the pain. Mother never attended a PTA meeting or met with my patient's teachers, and would spend weekends with her younger children's father, leaving my adolescent patient alone. She did not want her daughter to go away to college, because she needed her help at home, to take care of the children, to take care of the house. Through employment and loans the patient not only paid for four years of college, but sent money home to her mother. Unable to participate in social and extracurricular activities, my patient's college experience was a lonely one. While these incidents may not have been devastating, when the patient brought her mother to a session I saw from what her devastation arose. Mother set with us for a while, but in some way was not present: she could not look at me directly, and was unable to relate.

Though this mother's malattunement to my patient was devastating, the mother's treatment by *her* mother had been even more abusive. That mother, the patient's grandmother, failed to feed her child to such a degree she had to be hospitalized several times for malnutrition. The grandmother would tell one of her sons to beat my patient's mother, his sister, and he would comply, once breaking her arm. Neglect of my patient's mother reached a level that finally led authorities to remove her from her home, which they did when she was 11. She was placed in foster care, where, according to the patient's mother, she became a "slave".

The only place I have read of such violence in a home—though I know there are other instances—has been of slavers' behavior towards slaves. This is a Southern family, and given their poverty and social circumstances it is almost certain their ancestors had been slaves. And the probability is equally high that this grandmother had been the object of abuse. It is clear that her child's very being was anathema to her, that as far as she was concerned the child's feelings were of absolutely no significance, and that therefore she would never nurture, or contain this child. This, I maintain, is the void of which Gerson speaks, a void which holds affects, in this instance, of hatred and rage so injurious they are akin to death. In fact, my patient's aunts, the mother's sisters, have told the mother she would not have survived had she remained at home.

Another daughter, also mistreated by the patient's grandmother, left home but returned some time later with a child. This child was abused by both her mother and grandmother, and committed suicide at 16.

Both the patient's mother and the mother of the child who committed suicide are dark-skinned, which occasioned much of their mother's hostility. The designation of Africans as "blacks" has a long and complex history, and it is clear that the use of the term to connote something negative began long before discovery of the New World, as did its association with slavery (Davis, 2006).

Jordan (1968) cites a sixteenth-century English dictionary which defined black as dirty, soiled, evil, associated with death, etc. It is a term ripe with meaning, and given its application to *us*, it is hardly surprising we introjected those connotations. In the 1960s many of us sought to reverse the associations related to blackness with respect to African Americans: there were films, discussion groups, campaigns to get newspapers to cease their habitual identification of "Negro" in instances where its purpose seemed only to reinforce our "badness". The use of "black" as a term replacing Negro was one of the group's objectives, and its present acceptability is evidence of some success. However, the term's connotations are so deeply enculturated, and its significance for us so powerful, I wonder if it can ever become neutral.

Transmission

Until writing this chapter I had thought the process of traumatic transmission unfolds in the same manner as do all intersubjective phenomena, i.e., in the minute and molar, repetitive, verbal and nonverbal behaviors that constitute intersubjectivity. The way in which a child is held, the inflection of a verbal communication, the mother's expression as she peers over the crib in which her infant lies crying—can convey "your feelings matter to me—*you* matter to me—and I am that place where you can bring your pain and thereby be soothed". But a mother's repeated indifference to a toddler's falls, prohibition of disappointment when a long-awaited picnic is canceled by rain, convey your feelings *don't* matter—experienced by the child as y*ou* don't matter—and given her significance and magnitude, the wound to the child is severe.

As I wrote, however, I kept coming up against *voids, absences*—the parent's inability to give what was needed because the requisite emotional capacity did not exist. Whether it was my father, the mother of my subjugated, deadened patient, or the father of the patient who had "wack attacks"—all of these parents lacked what they had not been given. And Gerson (2009) and others hold that in some manner, this absence is transmitted to children, as it had been transmitted to them.

At times I have thought, "How can you talk about transmission of nothing? There is nothing to *carry*". Nothing except the parent's anguish, experienced as a child. What the child *does* receive, then, are the affects of this terrible nothingness, which, of course, is not nothing at all.

Bibliography

Atwood, G. & Stolorow, R. (2014). *Structures of Subjectivity*. London and New York, NY: Routledge.

Bandura, A. (2001). Social Cognitive Theory: An Agentic Perspective. *Annual Review of Psychology*, 52, 1–26.

Brandchaft, B. (1994). To Free the Spirit From Its Shell. In R. A. Stolorow, *The Intersubjective Perspective* (pp. 57–76). Northvale, NJ: Jason Aronson.

Cassidy, J. (1999). The Nature of the Child's Ties. In J. Cassidy & P. R. Shaver (Eds.), *Handbook of Attachment: Theory, Research, & Clinical Applications* (pp. 3–20). New York, NY: Guilford Press.

Davis, D. B. (2006). *Inhuman Bondage: The Rise and Fall of Slavery in the New World*. New York, NY: Oxford University Press.

Davoine, Francoise & Gaudilliere, Jean-Max. (2004). *Beyond History: Whereof One Cannot Speak, Thereof One Cannot Stay Silent*. New York, NY: Other Press.

Douglass, F. (1845/1987). Narrative of the Life of Frederick Douglass. In H. L. Gates, *The Classic Slave Narratives* (pp. 243–331). New York, NY: The Penguin Group.

Frankenberg, R. (1993). *The Social Construction of Whiteness: White Women, Race Matters*. Minneapolis, MN: University of Minnesota Press.

Gates, H. L. (2014) How Many Slaves Landed in the US? http://www.theroot.com./articles/history/2012/10/how-many-slaves-came-to-america-fact-vs-fiction.html

Gerson, S. (2009). When the Third is Dead: Memory, Mourning and Witnessing in the Aftermath of the Holocaust. *International Journal of Psychoanalysis*, 90, 6, 1341–1357.

Gump, J. P. (2010). Reality Matters: The Shadow of Trauma on African American Subjectivity. *Psychoanalytic Psychology* (1), 42–54.

Gump, J. (2014). Discovery and Repair: Discussion of the Article by Lynne Jacobs. *Psychoanalytic Inquiry*, 34, 759–765.

Jones, J. (1995). *Affects as Process: An Inquiry into the Centrality of Affect in Psychological Life*. Psychoanalytic Inquiry Book Series. New York, NY and London: Routledge.

Jordan, W. (1968). *White Over Black: American Attitudes Towards The Negro, 1550 – 1812*. Chapel Hill, NC: University of North Carolina Press.

Orange, D., Atwood, G. & Stolorow, R. (1997). *Working Intersubjectively*. Hillsdale, NJ: The Analytic Press.

Painter, N. (2010). *The History of White People*. New York, NY: W. W.Norton & Company.

Random House Dictionary of the English Language. (1966, 1967). New York, NY: Random House.

Socarides, D. D, & Stolorow, R. D, (1984). Affects and Self Objects, *The Annual of Psychoanalysis*, 12, 105–119.

Stolorow, R. & Atwood, G. (1992). *Contexts of Being*. Psychoanalytic Book Series, Vol. 12. Hillsdale, NJ: The Analytic Press,.

Stolorow, R., Atwood, G. & Brandchaft, B., Eds. (1994). *The Intersubjective Perspective*. Northvale, NJ: Jason Aronson, Inc.

Stolorow, R., Atwood, G. & Orange, D. (2002). *Worlds of Experience*. New York, NY: Basic Books.

Yetman, N. R. (2002). *When I was a Slave*. Mineola, NY: Dover Publications.

Chapter 10

Wounded stories

Alexander Etkind

From German memorials to Russian memoirs, one can trace a continuum of the cultural genres of mourning, but the contrasts are remarkably sharp. Though terror in Nazi Germany and Communist Russia both resulted in many millions of victims, their memories are different. The popular memory of the Holocaust boomed in the last years of the twentieth century on an industrial scale, but the popular memory of the Soviet terror has not advanced much since the times of the *Gulag Archipelago*.

The debate over the relationship between German Nazism and Soviet Communism has been a long and fierce one. Hannah Arendt's Cold-War era concept of totalitarianism, positing a metaphorical "common denominator" shared by the two regimes, was largely rejected by Western academics in the 1960s–80s, later embraced enthusiastically in Russia during the Gorbachev era, and has been largely resurrected in the Western scholarship of the new century. However, many Western thinkers, from Freud to Habermas and Derrida, have emphatically rejected the notion that these two regimes should be viewed as symmetrical.[1] In this chapter, I look at the response that one of the most important Western philosophers, Jacques Derrida, gave to this problem, and then proceed to the Russian cultural scene which looks different, I believe, after reading Derrida.

Derrida's silence

In 1981, Derrida was arrested in socialist Prague and spent two days in jail. Horrified by the experience, he saw no end to the Soviet domination of Eastern and Central Europe: "this barbarism could last for centuries".[2] He used the same popular label for the Soviet gulag, which he said was "at least equal to the Nazi barbarity".[3] However, Derrida remained faithful to the "specters of Marx"; crucially, he has described this faithfulness as a kind of grieving and haunting. In *Specters of Marx*, he presents this mourning for the spirit of communism as global and interminable, so that it amounts to what he calls a "geopolitical melancholy".

"We are heirs of Marxism, even before wanting or refusing to be, and like all inheritors, we are in mourning".[4] How can we understand this chain of metaphors? If it is true that we are heirs of Marxism, what we are mourning for? As Derrida repeatedly showed, metaphors are always pregnant with meaning, whether they work or not. Derrida's statement may refer to a particular victim of Marxism, who is not mentioned here though "we are in mourning", or, alternatively, it might mean that he is mourning the loss of his belief in Marxism, which is also not mentioned here, because "we are heirs". Derrida's statement could also combine both meanings, which corresponds to the condition of double mourning. This uneasy alternative finds illumination in Derrida's reminiscences about the leading Marxist philosopher, Louis Althusser. A tragic figure whose mature life started with imprisonment in a German POW camp and led to psychotic delusion and murder, Althusser was a long-time member of the French Communist Party. It was precisely in 1980—the year to which Derrida dates his own "apocalyptic" turn—that Althusser strangled his wife and was found mentally unfit to stand trial. Althusser would never recover his sanity, and Derrida has described his experience as he tried to care for his friend.[5]

Historian and psychoanalyst Elisabeth Roudinesco gives a striking interpretation of Althusser's ailment as "the melancholy of revolution".[6] She believes it to be similar to "a subjective collapse, a plunge into madness" that many went through, she states, after the French Revolution and its Terror. Conversing with Derrida about their mutual friend, Althusser, Roudinesco presents melancholy as an "invariant" of post-revolutionary situations. Following this logic, Roudinesco explains that "when an entire generation of communists were faced with the disaster of real socialism", they were "forced to mourn" their ideal, or "succumb to melancholy".[7]

Explicating the spirit of post-revolutionary melancholia, Derrida substitutes "ontology", a central term of traditional philosophy, with "hauntology", a science of specters and an art of talking to them. He feels that hauntology is the proper approach to Marxism, a ghost that was exorcized after the fall of the Soviet Union and the Berlin Wall, but continues its stalking and warning; he also emphasizes the ghostly metaphors of some crucial texts by Marx, most importantly the *Communist Manifesto* (1848) with its opening line, "A specter is haunting Europe—the specter of communism. All the powers of old Europe have entered into a holy alliance to exorcise this specter."[8] An inheritor, Derrida speaks more often about specters of Marx than about the ghosts of those who died for or because of Marxism; however, his hauntology embraces all these multi-natural spirits. In Colin Davis' formula, "hauntology is part of an endeavor to keep rising the stakes of literary study, to make it a place where we can interrogate our relation to the dead, examine the elusive identities of the living, and explore the boundaries between the thought and the unthought".[9] This ambitious endeavor also entails new ways of exploring the relations between the past, the present, and the future.

Inabilities to mourn

In the 1980s, the question of the incomparability of the Nazi crimes launched a fierce discussion in Germany, which is remembered as the "*Historikerstreit*" or the "Historians' Dispute". The dispute was sparked by a controversial statement by the philosopher Ernst Nolte, in which he emphasized the historical fact that the practices of state terror, such as concentration camps, had been developed in the Soviet Union earlier than in Germany and that German socialists knew of them well before the Nazis came to power, thus suggesting the direct influence of the Soviets upon the Nazis. The philosopher Jürgen Habermas found that these arguments entailed an unacceptable "historicization of the Holocaust" which, he argued, served to relieve the burden of historical guilt.

In Russia, this has not always been the case. While any comparison between the Soviet Union and Nazi Germany was a taboo during the Soviet period, Vasily Grossman in his *Life and Fate* produced a convincing analysis of resemblances, differences, and interactions between these two systems. Written in the 1950s but read in Russia only in the 1990s, this monumental novel unfolded, along with Solzhenitsyn's *The Gulag Archipelago*, as a credible and responsible history decades before academic historians approached the subject. After the collapse of the Soviet Union, a former member of the Politburo of its Communist Party, Aleksandr Yakovlev, characterized the Soviet regime in terms which alluded to the German parallel: "It was full-scale fascism of the Russian type. Our tragedy is that we have not repented." Yakovlev chaired the Presidential Commission for the Rehabilitation of the Victims of Political Repressions; as he knew well, "rehabilitation" was far from being synonymous with repentance. A founder of the Memorial Society, Veniamin Iofe wrote that the "chaos of speculations" about the Soviet past works like "a smoke-screen" which masks the problem of "evaluating the Soviet period of Russian history in terms as clear as those used for evaluating Nazi Germany."[10] Iofe obviously wanted the Russia of the 1990s to produce as "clear" a vision of its violent past as Germany had managed to do.

Several major factors should be taken into account in comparing the state of the German memory of National Socialism to the Russian memory of Soviet Socialism. First, the communist regime in Russia lasted much longer than the Nazi regime in Germany. Repairing the damage will probably hence require more time. In addition, Russia is less distant from the collapse of its Soviet state than Germany is from the collapse of its Nazi state. Since the Soviet regime lasted for seven decades, including at least three decades of terror, the concept of generation is less useful here than in the studies of the Holocaust survivors and their descendants. In post-Stalinist Russia, mourning was suspended for several decades, which included an abortive mourning period during Khrushchev's Thaw. Second, the Soviet victims were significantly more diverse than the Nazi victims; their descendants are more dispersed and in some cases, have competing interests, which creates multiple memory conflicts in the post-Soviet space. Third, Germany's post-war transformation was forced upon it by military defeat and occupation, while Russia's post-Soviet transformation was a political choice. No occupation force ruled Russia; it has continuously ruled itself. Instead of a Marshall Plan, the international support for the post-Soviet transition was remarkably inconsistent. Finally, there are substantial differences when it comes to the subjective experiences of victimization and mourning among the victims of both regimes and their descendants.

Decades ago, the French-Russian historian Mikhail Geller pinpointed the crucial difference here in a strong statement from his introduction to the first edition of Varlam Shalamov's *Kolyma Tales*:

> Kolyma is a twin of Hitler's death camps. But it is also different . . . The difference is that in Hitler's death camps, the victims knew why they were killed . . . Those who died in the Kolyma or other Soviet camps, died bewildered.[11]

If the Nazi theory of racial purity was implemented with consistency, the application of the Soviet theory of class warfare was more arbitrary. Most of those Jews and Gypsies who died in the Nazi camps agreed with their gaolers that they were Jews or Gypsies (though of course they did not agree that this should be cause to kill them). In contrast, most of those kulaks, saboteurs, and enemies of the people who died in the Soviet camps disagreed with their gaolers that they were kulaks, saboteurs, and enemies of the people. Some of them hated "enemies of the people" just as much as their gaolers did. In the Stalinist camps, many political prisoners shared the principles of their perpetrators but clung to the belief that in their personal cases, they had been mistakenly identified. In Nazi camps, on the other hand, the typical victim did not question his identification (e.g., as a Jew), but objected to the general reasons for his persecution.

Comparing the Russian and German memory of terror is like comparing two individuals at divergent points in the life cycle: an adolescent and an old man. In order to grasp their actual difference, one needs to imagine the old man in his younger years. Marking the end of the Nazi regime in 1945 and the end of the Soviet regime in 1991, we must judge the current state of Russian memory against German memory as it was documented in the 1960s. Germans had already experienced the Nuremberg trials (1945–46) and the Frankfurt Auschwitz Trials (1963–65). In Russia, an attempt to try the Communist Party failed in 1992. Germans began to open memorials and museums on the sites of camps in the 1960s; Russians started opening memorials in the 1990s. But in the 1960s, complaints about "collective amnesia" and "silencing the catastrophe" were probably as typical in Germany as they were in Russia over the last two decades.

The electorate in the graves

A political theory of mourning might be built upon the famous dictum of Edmund Burke, who in his polemics against the ideas of the French Revolution, claimed that the social contract "becomes a partnership not only between those who are living, but between those who are living, those who are dead, and those who are to be born". Different generations, living and dead, are partners in this contract which links "lower with higher natures [. . .] the visible and invisible world". More common in mystical contexts than in political ones, these concerns with the past and the dead were similarly theorized by Walter Benjamin, who wrote, "There is a secret agreement between past generations and the present one".[12] Disappointed with both the failure of revolution in Germany and its success in Russia,

Benjamin revived Burke's ideas. The same post-revolutionary formula inspired Derrida in his *Specters of Marx*, though Burke does not feature in its Index: no ethics or politics, writes Derrida, is just that does not recognize respect for those others who "are already dead or not yet born", and no justice is possible without responsibility "before the ghosts of those who are not yet born or who are already dead".

In the 1990s, when the Memorial Society discussed the forms of its political involvement in Russia's tortured transformation, one of its leaders, Veniamin Iofe, used to repeat: "Our electorate is there, in the graves".[13] Rejecting the direct participation of the Memorial in political elections, he proclaimed the unique role of the past in the post-catastrophic politics. Iofe was a physicist by training and probably never read Burke, but he knew the relevance of the "contract with the dead". A Soviet-era dissident and ex-prisoner, he also knew the affinity between memory and power.

Scholars tend to grumble about the condition of memory in contemporary Russia. Many speculate about collective nostalgia and cultural amnesia, or observe the "cold" character of the memory of Soviet terror.[14] Yet this notion of a deficit or crisis of popular historical knowledge in Russia does not reflect the current state of affairs and needs qualification. In fact, far from demonstrating an outright denial or forgetting of the Soviet catastrophe, the vast majority of Russians are well aware of their country's recent history. It is not historical knowledge that is at issue, but its interpretation. Sociological surveys reveal a complex picture of a people who retain a vivid memory of the Soviet terror but are divided in their interpretation of this memory. This interpretation inevitably depends upon the schemas, theories, narratives, and myths that people receive from their scholars, artists, and politicians. Many Russians explain the Soviet terror as an exaggerated but rational response to actual problems, which confronted the country at the time. These people believe that the terror was necessary for the survival of the nation, its modernization, industrialization, victory in the war, etc. In Holocaust studies, interpretations of this kind are called "redemptive narrative"; as Lawrence Langer has shown convincingly, the need for such redemption obstructs a sensible, "deep" connection to the catastrophic past.[15] Sociological polls reflect the massive spread of the need for a redemptive understanding of the past in contemporary Russia. However, the same polls say that the overwhelming majority of Russians and other post-Soviets are quite well aware of the crimes, misery, and "repressions" that remain memorable parts of the Soviet period. The polls, however, do not tell us about the substance of the historical truths and myths that the public believes in. Nor do they tell us why the public believes in the truth of some myths. They do not tell us who creates myths, mixes them with truths, and defines their changing boundaries.

No consensus on the crucial issues of historical memory has been reached in twenty-first-century Russia. Reflecting the moving equilibrium between the competing forces of politics, culture, and time, accepted definitions of what is "right" and "healthy" in the memory of the Soviet past shift with every new generation. While the state is led by former KGB officers who are no more interested in apologizing for the past than they are in fair elections in the present, the struggling civil society and the intrepid reading public are possessed by the unquiet ghosts of the Soviet era. But the circular time of post-catastrophic experience conflates uneasily with the linear time of history.[16] Whatever the scale of victimization, mourning remains a personal matter, but collective rituals and cultural artifacts are critical for the process. Sharing sorrow with the community, burial rituals prevent mourning from developing into melancholy. Crystals of memory, monuments keep the uncanny where it belongs, in the grave. The anthropologist Katherine Verdery asserts that "in many human communities, to set up right relations between living human communities and their ancestors depends critically on proper burials". Though it is never easy to learn which relations are "right", wrong relations are universally believed to be unfair to the dead and dangerous to the living.[17] In the post-Soviet economy of memory, where the losses are massive and the monuments in short supply, the dead return as the undead.

Having distinguished between two forms of cultural memory, the hardware and the software in Russian memory and mourning, I see the proliferation of a third form, which is impossible to reduce to the first two. I am referring to ghosts, spirits, vampires, dolls, and other manmade and man-imagined simulacra that carry the memory of the dead.[18] Usually, ghosts live in texts; sometimes, they inhabit cemeteries and emerge from monuments. Most often, ghosts visit those whose dead have not been properly buried. Texts are symbolic, while ghosts are iconic: as signs, ghosts possess a visual resemblance to the signified; in contrast to monuments, texts and ghosts are ephemeral; and in contrast to texts and monuments, ghosts are uncanny. These ghostly components of memory deserve a detailed analysis and close reading.[19]

Debt to the dead

When the literary scholar Andrei Siniavsky came home from the strict regime camp where he had served six years (1965–1971), he felt as though he had been split into pieces:

> And I began to weep . . . not for my lost youth but because of the *ridge*, as I called it, that had suddenly been erected in my mind, splitting me into two halves, into a *before* and an *after* my exit from behind the barbed wire, as though foreseeing how difficult it would be to return from there to people and what a chasm now lay between us and them.[20]

Siniavsky's major philological works were all written or conceived in the camp, and these works both reflected his camp experience and mourned other victims of the Soviet terror. Following Soviet culture through to its final stages and beyond, Siniavsky's critical and scholarly works deserve consideration on a par with his literary fiction, which has received more attention.[21] In both its quality and quantity, Siniavsky's camp output is remarkable, but not entirely unique. There are deep analogies to Siniavsky's camp oeuvre in the works of other authors who also spent years in camp or exile. They feature the unrestrained, radical "theses that sharply contradicted the conventional wisdom", which one of these ex-convicts, Dmitry Likhachev, believed to be characteristic of the writings that were produced in the gulag.[22] It has become traditional to distinguish several strands in the Soviet scholarship and criticism: official, émigré, and dissident. I believe that camp criticism represented an additional, separate and original strand of twentieth-century Russian scholarship.

Siniavsky's novella, *Liubimov* (1963), presents the well-known events of Russian revolutionary history as a series of miracles, ghostly apparitions, and collective hallucinations. Lenya, a little man in a provincial town, receives a revelation that gives him the power to hypnotize the local population. He confiscates all property in Liubimov, institutes round-the-clock surveillance over citizens, and organizes their collective labor. Supported by the hypnotically induced enthusiasm of the masses, his regime lasts until everyone, the leader and the masses, has exhausted their transformative energies. Curiously, Lenya received his hypnotic skills in the local library, where he borrowed an old mystical book; its author, a mid-nineteenth-century Freemason, visits the library as a ghost. The librarian, a hybrid character who is sometimes under Lenya's hypnoses and sometimes possessed by the nobleman's ghost, narrates the whole story. The Soviet government attacks the rebellious Liubimov, but Lenya is able to hypnotize its spies and soldiers. Lenya's rival and prototype, Lenin, is presented as a werewolf. The Liubimov citizens take the waters of the local river for champagne and Lenya for a dictator, but they feel happy only for so long as the hypnosis lasts. In the meantime, Lenya marries the local beauty. It then becomes clear that he is more interested in men than women, and so he turns a Soviet agent into his closest friend. The story ends when an Orthodox priest prays the Masonic ghost back into his grave, Lenya loses his power, and Soviet tanks raze Liubimov to the ground. An attempt to deconstruct the improbable course of Russian history by magical means, the novella anticipates many subsequent efforts of the writers who would become known in the 1980s.

Predating *One Hundred Years of Solitude* by Gabriel García Márquez (1967), Siniavsky's *Liubimov* and Daniel's *Moscow* share with this masterpiece of Magical Realism its complex narrative structure and free-wheeling experimentation with history. Siniavsky and Daniel are the two most important predecessors of leading post-Soviet authors such as Vladimir Sharov, Vladimir Sorokin, and Dmitry Bykov, who would continue their experiments with violence, libraries, and history. Most importantly, one could read both of these unusual texts, *Liubimov* and *Moscow* as Victims' Balls, imaginary rituals of mimetic mourning that would have run amok had they been realized. But can we be so sure that they were never realized? There are details in the life stories and court trials of Daniel, Siniavsky, Brodsky, and even Vysotsky that make me think that, with all the ambivalence that one can imagine, these figures provoked their persecutions and imprisonment through their actions, which we might read as a form of mimetic mourning. After the collapse of its major structures in 1953–1956, the gulag became a sacred place, but reaching this destination required a very serious effort. The undertaking of the pilgrimage to the gulag was a task for the writer, the priest of the emerging culture of mourning. Some made the pilgrimage as tourists, and brought back souvenirs from the mass graves for their writing desks; some made the pilgrimage by turning themselves into prisoners—the way of mimetic self-sacrifice; some imagined these visits for their readers.

Siniavsky's novel, *Goodnight!*, describes his return from the camp to Moscow as an expulsion from home and a loss of vision. He compared himself to a boy who had completed his prison term and was now supposed to go home, but could not bear to leave, so he wept and begged to be let back into the camp; the guard drove him away, but he kept coming back again and again, unable to bring himself to set off for home. There is a meaningful resemblance between Siniavsky's self-documented desire to return to the camp and the story which Bitov tells in his *Pushkin House* of the ex-convict who does return to the site of the camp, to die there

After his release, Siniavsky found that he needed to wear eye-glasses. He understood this loss of vision as a symbol of a deeper regress that he experienced when he returned home. After being so prolific in the camp, he found himself unable to write after his return to Moscow; he overcame this block only when he moved further on, to Paris. He wrote that through his glasses, one of his eyes contemplated the alien Moscow life, while the other eye looked back to the camp. Life in the camp was "more complete and more inspiring" than life in Moscow. Even the prison, the worst place of all, had a "style and rhythm" he never saw again, either in Russia or abroad—"frightening, attractive, and joyful".[23]

After decades of state terror, the camps of the sixties were full of ghosts. With a deliberate ambiguity, Siniavsky wrote to his wife: "Everything here is a bit fantastic, even flowers and encounters . . . The sun is lower on the horizon, and therefore the shadows are longer . . . My neighbor is spectral, we slept and ate together, and suddenly it turned out that he is a specter" (2/62). Those who were released from the camp also felt illusory or hallucinatory, but for a different reason: "they have immediately become spectral and unearthly, as if they were dead" (2/169). Everything was ghostly because of the camp's boredom and loneliness; everything was haunted because of its history and symbolism. After liberation, Siniavsky himself felt like a specter issuing from the camp: "Leaving prison is like being re-born after death .. All that remains is a naked point of view, so you feel like a ghost visiting this world."[24]

The favorite subjects of Siniavsky's studies—Pushkin, Gogol, and sectarians—were also, at their best and most creative moments, suspended in this intermediary, reversible state between life and death. Sveshnikov portrayed this condition in his memorable images; Siniavsky depicted it in his book, *In the Shadow of Gogol*:

In the "transitory condition", as Gogol put it (and all his work was like a transitory, loose swing between life and death) . . . his personality split into some kind of multitude, which existed on different levels of being and consciousness, dying and resurrecting itself daily, and even from somewhere beyond the grave still reaching back to life, and weeping, and threatening, and arguing with compatriots.

(2/189)

Gogol "was dying all his life"; Gogol "encompassed within himself the impassable gap between the living and the dead"; Gogol lived "in the coffin of his tired, almost unresponsive flesh". Such was also the life of the typical inmates of the camps, the goners. Siniavsky escaped their fate but Sveshnikov had been one of these soon-to-be-dead before the camp doctor saved him. It was in their shadow—in the shadow of Gogol—that Siniavsky wrote the camp letters that contained his future books. From the vanguard position of the goner, Gogol manifested "a striking ability to reason and control . . . seeing more and farther than normal vision can see".[25]

Siniavsky's wife sent him a book about vampires and a collection of Gothic novels in Russian translation. Sectarians in the camp gave him mystical manuscripts to read. But none of this was ever enough; Siniavsky's "dream of reading about ghosts" (2/165) remained unsatisfied, and he asked for more. Calling the time of his youth "the period of late, mature, and blooming Stalinism", he remembered "craziness, plots, horrors . . . ghouls, vampires, which still do not let me sleep", and also the "atmosphere of the black mass, a dog's wedding, and howling from beyond the grave."[26] These youthful motifs would often find a place in Siniavsky's texts. Their poetics are monstrous, but the author saw it as resulting from the historical reality in which he lived and worked. "Monsters are just as universal as the little devils that alcoholics see in their dreams," Siniavsky wrote (1/356-7)—in other words, not universal at all, but rather specific to the sinner and his sins. Besides this clinical awareness, there was not much to rely on for a child of Stalinism who wished to stroll with the ghosts.

Uninvited guests

Siniavsky's conclusions had always been extreme, but it was the brutal experience of the camp that prompted him to produce a more literal interpretation of the heretical and monstrous than either the Russian Symbolist poets or their scholarly heirs, the Soviet semioticians, ever dared to perform. In a way that resembled Walter Benjamin, whom he never read, Siniavsky interpreted the great texts of the Russian poetic tradition—Pushkin's "Prophet", Lermontov's "Demon", Gogol's "A Terrible Vengeance", as memories of religious rituals. "Telling fairytales required dedication and extreme caution . . . Violating these conditions brought disaster in its wake, even the death of the storyteller . . . The figure of the storyteller was surrounded by mystery, suffering, and omniscience" (2/385).

The camp experience stimulated the writing of ghost stories and helped to make visible the monstrous aspects of classical texts. In Siniavsky's camp and post-camp writings, Pushkin was a vampire; the romantic Russian *troika* was harnessed to the devil; Gogol oscillated between a goner and a revenant; and Soviet civilization was monstrous. Siniavsky's wife made a distinction between death in the camp and death in civil life: there people die, in the camp they croak (*dokhnut*). Mandelstam, for example, croaked, she said.[27] Since life in the camp was not human life, death there was not human death. The difference was social and also temporal. In civil life, death is a boundary, an instantaneous turn from one condition to another. There is no grey zone here. It is different in the camp, where there is nothing but the grey zone. "Dying alive is worse than death", writes Siniavsky in his essay on Shalamov. "Death in Kolyma was dispersed in time and space. Here death was drawn out over many years and thousands of kilometers." A gradual loss of life turned people into "building material with which the builders could do whatever they liked". Whether this was life or death, it was not a human condition. "Shalamov writes as though he were dead", states Siniavsky.[28] In his Siberian servitude, Dostoevsky experienced the same "passage through death."[29] Life in the camp was worse than death for two reasons, writes Siniavsky. The first reason was the victim's pain, the second was survivor's guilt: "in the condition of Kolyma, every life was egotism, a sin, the murder of one's neighbor".[30] People create art, wrote Siniavsky from the camp, "for the sake of overcoming death, but also in rapt anticipation of death" (1/64). Art is "just a histrionic one-man-show in the face of death" (2/377). Or—for the unluckiest—of croaking.

In light of Shalamov's and Siniavsky's witnessing, bare life of the goners should more properly be called monstrous life. Life in the camp—monstrous life between life and death—knows only the movement towards death. This is why, in the camp, Pushkin was construed as a ghoul, Gogol was imagined alive in his coffin, and the neighbors looked like ghosts: it was the camp. In 1974 in Paris, Siniavsky claimed that the camp was the most important theme of Russian literature of the time. "The Russian writer's heart doesn't burn ... for agricultural or industrial themes right now. He is concerned with other themes: how people get put away, where they're sent into exile, how exactly (it's interesting, after all!) they're shot in the back of the head."[31] Russian books have always been written in blood. An author is the writing dead. The literary form has a shape of coffin. This is how Siniavsky distributed his monstrous metaphors. His picture of "the literary process in Russia" built on his recent strolls with ghosts: "The camp theme is leading and central today ... Now all of Russia is howling in the House of the Dead".[32] In this focus, Siniavsky was different even from his beloved Rozanov. A model for modern Russian writers, Rozanov was always eager to explain human actions as manifestations of sexuality. In contrast, Siniavsky understood even the sexual act itself in the context of death and memory. Describing the annual visits his wife made to the camp, he rendered the rhythm and meaning of the sex act as an act of memory: "Remember before the end. Until the end. Remember. Remember. Understand and remember."[33]

The voices of the dead speaking through the lips of the half-dead—this is how Siniavsky saw the Russian literature of his time. "And they're moving, they're on the move now. As long as I live, as long as we all live—they will go on and on".[34] They were prisoners at the gates of the camp, and they were either leaving the camp or trying to find their way back to it, we never know which. For Siniavsky, the author is a medium who speaks with both the dead and the living, on behalf of both. "The living owe a debt to the dead." This is why the Russian author feels most at home in a prison or a madhouse, said Siniavsky. "He sits there quietly ... and he rejoices: here is my story!" Like Gogol to the cemetery, Siniavsky was drawn to the camps.

One can (also) feel the swift evolution of the popular style of historicizing by watching and comparing several Russian films, starting from the pre-post-Soviet *Zero City* by Karen Shakhnazarov (1988). In the course of the film, the narrative gradually shifts from an anti-bureaucratic comedy to a fable about the grasping power of the past. The protagonist is a typical Soviet man, an unambitious engineer who comes from Moscow to a provincial factory on a business trip. Screened as a drama of misrecognition, the story focuses on the investigation of a local scandal that was suppressed in the 1960s but leads to a suicide in the 1980s. Irresistibly drawn into this provincial story, the protagonist finds himself unable to escape. A key setting for this imprisonment is the local historical museum, where the engineer is presented with a past that feels more lively and consequential than his present has ever been. He ends up stuck in the museum, under the sway of a monotonous, pedantic historian who presents this Soviet Everyman with an astonishing panoply of pictures of the past in the form of group statues composed of living people. Full of tricks, conspiracies, and outright hallucinations that are all presented as apparitions of the past, the film leaves the after-taste of a mystery that has not been resolved by its creators.

In the spirit of melancholy, *Zero City* combines an ecstatic fascination with the great but horrible past with a vague anxiety about the future. Conveying expert knowledge but zero sympathy for the late-Soviet present, this film still lacked the staple feature of post-Soviet cinema: hostile, mystical beasts that operate among humans and interfere with their present. In contrast to hyper-historical *Zero City, Night Watch* and its sequel, *Day Watch* (2004, 2006), demonstrate the post-Soviet infatuation with magic in a deliberately abstract, ahistorical context. Based on the bestselling trilogy by Sergei Lukianenko, a psychiatrist from Kazakhstan who has made himself into one of the most popular post-Soviet authors, these films present an enormous taxonomy of immortal creatures. Vampires and other supernatural beasts rule over Russians, and live in their midst. Humans are entirely deprived of self-control, autonomy, and political life in this world. As in a camp, these Muscovites have been reduced to bare life, and essentially fulfill the role of the vampires' cattle (the vampires in the film prefer human blood but will settle for pigs' blood if necessary). Actual politics are deployed by creatures of a higher order than vampires and humans. These creatures are immortal and powerful but otherwise look like humans. The origins of their conflict are projected back to medieval Europe in one episode, and to the Asia of Genghis Khan in another. As in historical debates between contemporary Russian intellectuals, the roots of the current problems are presented as lost and found in the most distant time and spaces, but not in current or recent Russian politics. There is not a word in this movie about Stalin or the Soviet Union. The contemporary commoners, all of whom are potential victims of vampires, are juxtaposed against noble warriors whose moments of glory and sources of conflicts are all in the past. What matters is not happening here and now; it all happened in the past. The past, which is imagined as grand and foreign, determines the actual, dismal present. While the contemporary rulers are of alien and metaphysical origins, the vampires are local and earthly. The vampires represent, as they do in Slavic folklore, the unburied dead, while the remarkable face of their leader reflects a free play of Soviet shadows.[35] These films convey a static, irresolvable melancholy that risks slipping into paranoia. If vampires really ruled Russia, this is the worldview that they would disseminate among their human chattels to keep them subdued and passive. In the battle between light and dark forces, what is at stake is probably not the right to license vampires' bloodsucking activities, as *Night Watch* suggests. Inverting the film's metaphor, the only means of preventing the reproduction of vampires is to bury, acknowledge, and remember the dead.

In Tengiz Abuladze's film *Repentance* (1984), which is now a Soviet classic, the daughter of a victim digs up the corpse of the dictator. She goes on trial but does not repent: she would do it three hundred times over, she declares. It is not the corpse of the dictator that is uncanny in this film but the living dictator, as he is remembered or imagined by his former subjects. As in Sophocles' *Antigone*, the perpetually moving corpse begets new tragedies; in *Repentance*, it brings about the suicide of the dictator's grandson.[36] In *The Living* (2006, directed by Aleksandr Veledinsky), a Russian soldier of the Chechen War, Kir, is rescued by his comrades who are then themselves killed in action. On his way home from the war, Kir murders his officer and cheats on his fiancée. He does not care; he is possessed by the ghosts of his lost comrades, who come to him alive though other people do not see them. When Kir and his ghostly companions travel to Moscow, what they (and the viewers) actually see is the burial monument to Stalin near the Kremlin Wall. The movie ends with Kir's visit to an abandoned cemetery where he hopes to find his friends buried like heroes. While trying to find these graves, Kir dies; immediately, he joins the company of his ghostly fellows. The multiple tricks that the undead play with the living in this film force the viewer to suspect that the soldier was probably dead from the very beginning; perhaps all or a large part of what we see actually happened to his ghost.

These two films, *Repentance* and *The Living*, mark the start and the possible end of the post-Soviet transition, which may yet turn out to have been a false start and a dead end. In the 1980s, it seemed that the most important goal was to punish the dead dictator and in this way, to restore justice posthumously; 20 years later, the living were still struggling with the authorities, but their unburied dead were friends, not foes. There are enemies who are alive and deserve death, but there are also friends who are dead and need to be buried. Both films play on the uncanny effects of communication between the living and the dead; but while *Repentance* celebrates the change of generations, the trial of memory, and historical time, *The Living* deconstructs the meaning of death in an obsessive way that makes time cyclical and history irrelevant. Still hopeful for the future, *Repentance* argued for a new ethical order that would include dead corpses in its scope. Self-censoring any sign of hope, *The Living* showed the ghostly nature of post-catastrophic consciousness, which obscures the very difference between the living and the dead. Here, the post-Soviet trial of the dead gives way to a new Russian communion and mingling with the dead.

Having taught the relevance of ghosts to the interpretative community of his readers, Derrida does not offer much help in understanding their nature, taxonomy, or life cycle. As some critics have mentioned, his ghosts are not the same as the sophisticated phantoms of Nicolas Abraham and Maria Torok, which keep the secrets of the past and transmit them, in eternally encrypted form, from generation to generation. Derrida's ghosts could reveal a secret if they wished, but they do not necessarily do that, and the reason behind their existence is different from this conspiratorial knowledge. "It is in the name of *justice*" that Derrida speaks about the ghosts, and not in the name of knowledge. But this is a special kind of justice, one that brings the living and the dead together in a single ghostly equation. As for Burke, for Derrida "present existence . . . has never been the condition . . . of justice". Theirs is the justice of relations between the living and the dead. It needs to be established "*through* but also *beyond* right and law",[37] though not beyond human comprehension, with its rhetorical devices such as ghosts. Practically speaking, this particular "justice", one of the most frequent concepts in Derrida's late writings, is the debt owed to the dead.

But it is also true that these debts before the dead can never be returned and this justice can never be established. I am sure that all our philosophers of mourning would agree with this thesis, which gives post-catastrophic mourning its interminable, melancholic character. Having granted these images—ghosts, debts, posthumous justice—all the metaphorical relevance they deserve, one still feels puzzled by them. How can we the living redeem our debt to the dead? What kind of justice are we talking about? Can we repay the ghosts? Do we have a currency that is convertible for this task? Can this toolkit of legal and financial metaphors provide any help in carrying out the work of mourning?

Derrida links his hauntology with the idea of retributive justice. In a post-catastrophic situation, we mourners live lives and die deaths that are incomparably better than those of our precursors. This is why to live with ghosts means "to live otherwise, and better. No, not better, but more justly."[38] This kind of justice does not require judiciary power, but it does need scholars. As the living and the undead grow more accustomed to each other, they develop an uneasy friendship that needs to be noticed, articulated, and recognized. As Derrida urged, the ghostly dimension of our lifeworld is permanent; we must "learn to live with ghosts." This is a departure from a folklore understanding of ghostly apparitions as consequences of improper burial rites, with the implicit promise that re-burial would send the ghosts safely back to their graves. Derrida does not wish this to happen as a general case, and I do not see it happening in Russia. In contrast to laying them to rest, learning to live with ghosts is an open-ended process, which generates the unpredictable and rich variety of Victim's Balls, memory events, and cultural innovations.

These mournful experiences need to be summarized, but I feel that justice is a poor concept for doing this work. In my view, ghosts need recognition rather than justice. There is no way to redistribute anything of value between the dead and the living; but there is a very real sense in which unjustifiable deaths can be recognized by the living. Ghosts demand recognition.

This chapter features excerpts from Chapter 6 (pp.111–133) and Chapter 10 (pp.196–219) of *Warped Mourning: Stories of the Undead in the Land of the Unburied* by Alexander Etkind. Copyright © 2013 by the Board of Trustees of the Leland Stanford Jr. University. All rights reserved. Reprinted by permission of Stanford University Press.

Notes

1 On Freud's thinking about the changing regime in Russia, see A. Etkind (1997). *Eros of the Impossible. The History of Psychoanalysis in Russia.* Boulder, CO: Westview. 225–27.
2 Derrida, *Specters of Marx*, 87; others sources give 1982 as the date for the arrest.
3 Jacques Derrida, Elisabeth Roudinesco (2004). *For What Tomorrow. A Dialogue*, trans. Jeff Rort. Stanford, CA: Stanford University Press. 82.
4 Derrida, *Specters of Marx*, 126, 67.
5 Derrida, Roudinesco. *For What Tomorrow,* 79.
6 Roudinesco compares Althusser to the protagonist of her book and a heroine of the French Revolution, Théroigne de Méricourt, whose descent into insanity coincided with the rise of the Terror that followed the revolution. Elisabeth Roudinesco (1992). *Madness and Revolution: The Lives and Legends of Théroigne de Méricourt.* London: Verso. This study of post-revolutionary melancholy was originally published in 1989, the year of the bicentenary of the French Revolution and also, the fall of the Berlin Wall.
7 Derrida and Roudinesco. *For What Tomorrow*, 76.

Julie Fedor drew my attention to a fascinating detail: the first English translation by Helen MacFarlane (1850) rendered this line as "A frightful hobgoblin stalks through Europe."; see e.g. "A Frightful Hobgoblin . . . ", DACH BLOG: The British Library's German, Austrian and Swiss Collections, 25 February 2010, accessed 8 January 2012, http://britishlibrary.typepad.co.uk/dach/2010/02/a-frightful-hobgoblin.html.
9 Colin Davis (2007). *Haunted Subjects: Deconstruction, Psychoanalysis and the Return of the Dead*. London: Palgrave Macmillan. 13.
10 Aleksandra Samarina's interview with Aleksandr Yakovlev, *Obshchaia gazeta*, 18 October 2001; V.V. Iofe, "Reabilitatisiia kak istoricheskaia problema", in his *Granitsy smysla* (St. Petersburg: Memorial, 2002), 7.
11 Mikhail Geller (1978). "Predislovie," in Varlam Shalamov, *Kolymskie Rasskazy*. London: Overseas Publications Interchange. 8–9; see also his pioneering book: Mikhail Geller (1974). *Kontsentratsionnyi mir i sovetskaia literature*. London: Overseas Publications Interchange.
12 Walter Benjamin (1968). "Theses on the Philosophy of History", in his *Illuminations*. New York, NY: Schocken Books. 254.
13 Irina Flige, personal communication, November 2002.
14 See e.g. Sarah E. Mendelson and Theodore P. Gerber (2005). "Soviet Nostalgia: An Impediment to Russian Democratization," *Washington Quarterly* 29, no. 1: 83–96; Maria Ferretti, "Rasstroistvo pamiati: Rossiia i stalinizm," accessed 14 December 2011, http://old.polit.ru/documents/517093.html; and Charles S. Maier (2001–2002). "Heißes und kaltes Gedachtnis. Uber die politische Halbwertszeit von Nazismus und Kommunismus," *Transit* 22 (Winter): 53–165. For a re-evaluation of this position, see Tatiana Zhurzhenko (2007). "The Geopolitics of Memory," *Eurozine*, 10 May 2007, accessed 14 December 2011, www.eurozine.com/articles/2007-05-10-zhurzhenko-en.html.
15 Lawrence Langer (1991). *Holocaust Testimonies: The Ruins of Memory*. New Haven, CT: Yale University Press.
16 For theoretical discussion of the temporality of collective trauma, see Jenny Edkins (2003). *Trauma and the Memory of Politics*. Cambridge: Cambridge University Press. Chap. 2.
17 Katherine Verdery (1999). *The Political Lives of Dead Bodies: Reburial and Postsocialist Change*. New York, NY: Columbia University Press. 42–43.
18 A proliferation of ghosts and zombies in high and popular cultures has been observed by scholars of post-socialist transformations in Poland, East Germany, Ukraine, and Russia. For a similar effect in South Africa after apartheid, see Jean and John Comaroff (2002). "Alien-Nation: Zombies, Immigrants, and Millenial Capitalism." *The South Atlantic Quarterly* 104/4: 779–805. While I am writing, the most recent example is a Cuban film, *Juan of the Dead*, described as "the blood-drenched tale of a slacker who decides to save the island from an invasion of cannibalistic zombies", though the film is also "scattered with allusions to traumatic moments in Cuba's recent history" (Victoria Burnett in *The New York Times*, 10 December 2011).
19 One scholar of German memory confronting similar problems has devised an approach which he calls "spectral materialism"; see Eric L. Santner (2006). *On Creaturely Life. Rilke, Benjamin, Sebald*. Chicago, IL: University of Chicago Press. 52.
20 Abram Tertz [Andrei Siniavskii] (1984). *Spokoinoi Nochi*. Paris: Sintaksis. 43.
21 Western works on Siniavsky tend to read him as an author of philosophical prose, who was able to transcend his cultural context; Margaret Dalton (1973). *Andrei Siniavskii and Julii Daniel. Two Soviet "Heretical" Writers*. Wurzburg: Jal-Verlag; Olga Matich (1989). "Spokojnioj noci. Andrej Sinjavskij's Rebirth as Abram Terc", *Slavic and East European Journal* 33, no. 1 (Spring); Stephanie Sandler (1992). "Sex, Death and Nation in the *Strolls with Pushkin* Controversy", *Slavic Review*, 51, no. 2 (Summer): 294–308; Catharine Theimer Nepomnyashchy (1995). *Abram Tertz and*

the Poetics of Crime. New Haven, CT and London: Yale University Press, and her "Andrei Donatovich Siniavsky (1925–1997)", *Slavic and East European Journal*, 42, no. 3 (1998): 368; Harriet Murav (1998). *Russia's Legal Fictions.* Ann Arbor, MI: University of Michigan; Walter F. Kolonosky (2003). *Literary Insinuations: Sorting out Siniavsky's Irreverence.* Lanham, MD: Lexington Books. Beth Holmgren was specifically interested in the pretexts and contexts of Siniavsky's fiction; see her "The Transfiguring of Context in the Work of Abram Tertz", *Slavic Review*, 50, no. 4 (Winter 1991): 965–77. On Siniavsky's non-fiction, see Tat'iana Ratkina (2010). *Nikomu ne zadolzhav: Literaturnaia kritika i esseistika A.D. Siniavskogo.* Moscow: Sovpadenie. The recently published massive collection of Siniavsky's camp letters provides new material for analysis: Andrei Siniavskii (2004). *127 pisem o liubvi*, 3 vols. Moscow: Agraf, cited below by volume and page number. See also Yulii Daniel' (2000). *"Ya vse sbivaius' na literaturu". Pism'a iz zakliucheniia. Stikhi.* Moscow: Memorial-Zven'ia.
22 Dmitrii Likhachev, *Vospominaniia*, 142.
23 *Ibid.*, 30, 40.
24 Tertz (1991). *Golos iz khora,* in his*: Sobranie sochinenii*, vol. 1. Moscow: Start. 664.
25 Tertz (2009). *V teni Gogolia.* Moscow: KoLibri. 8, 17, 19, 106.
26 Tertz, *Spokoinoi nochi*, 323, 325–6.
27 Mariia Rozanova (1992). "K istorii i geografii etoi knigi', *Voprosy literatury* 10: 156. In his article, "Literaturnyi protsess v Rossii", Siniavsky said the same of Mandelstam's death (184).
28 Siniavskii (1980). "O 'Kolymskikh rasskazakh' Varlama Shalamova. Srez materiala", in his (2003) *Literaturnyi protsess v Rossii.* Moscow: RGGU. 341.
29 Siniavskii, (1981). "Dostoevskii i katorga", in his *Literaturnyi protsess*, 334.
30 Siniavskii, "O 'Kolymskikh rasskazakh'", 339.
31 Siniavskii, "Literaturnyi protsess", in his *Literaturnyi protsess,* 179.
32 Ibid.
33 Tertz, *Spokoinoi nochi*, 192.
34 Tertz, Golos iz khora.
35 These films have been the subject of several studies: Stephen M. Norris draws analogies between these films' plotlines and actual events in Russian politics in his "In the Gloom: The Political Lives of Undead Bodies in Timur Bekmambetov's Night Watch", *KinoKultura* 16 (2007), accessed 14 December 2011, http://www.kinokultura.com/2007/16-norris.shtml; a glossy Russian volume demonstrates the "kulturologia" approach to these films and features essays by Boris Groys and Mikhail Ryklin (2006). In B. Kupriianov and M. Surkov (Eds.), *Dozor kak Simptom.* Moscow: Falanster.
36 Interestingly, the recent *Katyn* by Andrzej Waida (2007), which shows the slaughter of thousands of Polish officers by their Russian "allies" in 1940, also refers to Antigone. A female character struggles to bury her brother who was murdered by the Russians; to earn money for the tombstone, she sells her hair to a Warsaw theater which needs wigs for their production of *Antigone*; see A. Etkind et al., (2012). *Remembering Katyn.* Cambridge: Polity.
37 Derrida, *Specters of Marx*, 221.
38 Derrida, *Specters of Marx*, xviii.

Afterword

Sam Gerson

The ghostly occupies our imagination both as vexation and as salvation. In one sensibility there are the horrors of being inhabited by something, someone, some time, not our own. In another register, there is the welcoming relief of contact with that which was lost, never was, and may yet be. Ghosts as intrusive inhabitants and as anchoring attachments. Yet, whatever form they assume, the ghostly and the demonic remain enigmatic in their representation of our conflicted desires and fears.

Taking license from Laplanche's (1989) startling question: "What does the breast want from me?", we might ask "what does the ghost want from me?" A query that is perhaps even more enigmatic as ghosts and demons are forever skirting death, whereas the breast is shaping desire. The ghost seeks refuge from the void, while the breast sustains life. We are in the realms of Thanatos and Eros and as we traverse these domains we must also wonder how our own fear and desire create the frightening and alluring spirits. We must ask: "what do I want from the ghost?" And occupied with this query, we are wrapped in the bafflements of a double enigmatic signifier – what do the dead want from me and what do I want from the dead?

The editors of this volume suggest the conflicts that ensue from this enigmatic weave create an enduring sense of an empty core at the heart of one's being. This is the "absent presence" that may yield " . . . a kind of moral abdication, a deadness at the core of the soul that insists on not knowing" (p.3). We must imagine that the imperative to not know is secondary to exposure to experiences that defy comprehension, that destroy representation, and that leave one utterly bereft of an other who might mitigate the deadliness of a life stripped of passion and compassion. Contemporary literature offers many renditions of this tragic form of life – a ghostly existence poignantly captured in Eugene O'Neill's hallmark twentieth-century American drama *Long Day's Journey Into Night*. In this haunting play, all of the characters imagine that there might be salvation in a ghostly existence that offers a sanctuary from devilish punishment and demonic possession.

Consider too in this regard Samuel Beckett's *Waiting for Godot*. The abiding wish for a live presence that might release the protagonists Vladimir and Estragon from the claims of the dead is met also by the pain of traumatic experience and the seductions of absence. In a particularly poignant moment in their "conversation", the two lost characters search their own sensorium for some semblance of meaning while searching each other for a witnessing echo in the midst of their interminable wait. In the murmuring sounds of rustling leaves and whispering wind, they hear "all the dead voices" and wonder if and when the dead will ever be heard enough to rest. There are voices that do not speak in words; rather there are sounds, faint and persistent, that each receives sensorially and subjects to his own translation. The sounds of the dead that cannot rest without being heard, yet who communicate with those who cannot understand. Like ghosts or demons, they are the embodiment of a knowledge that cannot be known as they herald the unspeakable.

Beckett's work also reminds that what Estragon and Vladimir may have lost, and what they await, is not only an other, but also the possibility of maintaining a coherent and stable internal representation of a benign other in the face of unspeakable terror. A terror that sweeps through communal life leaving one bereft of faith in oneself, in an other, and in the future.

We all wish to leave a livable future for our descendants even while knowing the damaging and damaged nature of our social surround. The authors in this volume have offered us entry into the horrors we often wish to forget, or visit briefly, fearing that the dark vision will invade and contaminate our faith. Still, we are drawn toward this knowledge in the belief that our responsibilities to the other can only achieve enduring purpose when we are ourselves in communion with both Eros and Thanatos. And yet, we also know how those who are most engaged with bearing witness to the dehumanizations suffered daily are subject to their own debilitating loss of hope (e.g. the Holocaust authors Jean Amery, Paul Celan, and Primo Levi).

Walter Benjamin (1940) captured both the ethos and pathos of the imperative to speak of the trauma infiltrating all of our lives in his oft-noted passage entitled *The Angel of History* – an essay that was inspired by a painting created after World War I, in 1920, by Paul Klee titled "Angelus Novus".

> A (Paul) Klee painting named "Angelus Novus" shows an angel looking as though he is about to move away from something he is fixedly contemplating. His eyes are staring, his mouth is open, his wings are spread. This is how one pictures the angel of history. His face is turned toward the past. Where we perceive a chain of events, he sees one single catastrophe which keeps piling wreckage upon wreckage and hurls it in front of his feet. The angel would like to stay, awaken the dead, and make whole what has been smashed. But a storm is blowing from Paradise; it has got caught in his wings with such violence that the angel can no longer close them. The storm irresistibly propels him into the future to which his back is turned, while the pile of debris before him grows skyward. The storm is what we call progress.
>
> (p. 257, 1940)

I am always shaken when I read these lines - first because they were written shortly before Benjamin's death by suicide when his plan to escape Vichy France was thwarted at the Spanish border in the Pyrenees; and then by the image and words describing how the residue of destruction not only documents historical calamities, but becomes itself a force sowing a deadly future whose horror haunted his, and our, hope.

The insistent claims of our histories are most often relayed to us through the voice of an intimate member of our family and these are immeasurably magnified when the content of the address of the other is filled with the fragmented narrative and emotional sequella of trauma. These are horrors that enjoin us to create coherence from chaos and yet we are left occupied with a violence that defies knowledge, even as it demands to be known. As we know, the transmission of trauma across generations – in as much as trauma has created "zones of non-symbolization" (Levy, 2012) – includes being inhabited with the non-representable and the forces that destroyed representation. And from this destruction come the haunting questions: "What does the other's experience demand of me? Must I identify with their experience to ensure their survival in me? And in this quest, must I be traumatized as well?"

We are all born into the claims of history, family and community. Judith Butler (2004) captured this pervasive force when she wrote that " . . . what binds us morally has to do with how we are addressed by others in ways that we cannot avert or avoid; this impingement by the other's address constitutes us first and foremost against our will or, perhaps put more appropriately, prior to the formation of our will" (p.130). We are reminded here that from the first, all identifications carry the seeds of conflict as they originate from the other, from the past, from necessity and so constitute a confused ontology of the self. As Ferenczi (1909) noted "identification is an encounter with ghosts of the past". The essays of this book brought our awareness to identifications that are so filled with horror that we are left imagining that there is a residue within which even ghosts cannot survive. It is this void which pulls for an identification with irredeemable and unfathomable loss, losses that may eventuate in what Faimberg (2005), has termed "alienated identifications" – the unconscious incorporation and enactment of the dissociated and the disavowed.

This is the "absent presence", an identification with melancholic states wherein demons are embodiments of the melancholic spirit that saturate the subject to such an extent that even phantasy externalizations do not rid the self of absence. In such states there is a fracturing of continuity between self and others that leaves fissures in the individual's sense of the integrity of the world and of themselves; as one patient put it "I feel that there is a gaping hole at my core and my vitality constantly drains into this empty place". As there is a melancholic identification, but no mourning of loss, the absences create a never-ending necessity of contending with unrepresented experience and sensibility, and thus unlike mourning that which has been lost, absence yields unending anxiety that something essential for full life and vitality interminably eludes one (LaCapra, 2001).

Absence, rather than being a trauma that is transmitted from the past, might be better thought of as a trauma of not being able to forge connections across time and between past, present, and future. It is a trauma that often manifests in issues of identity confusion, social alienation, split loyalties, impotent love and rage, and a deep sense of discontinuity between external and internal life. We may capture an aspect of this by inverting Loewald's (1979) Oedipal trajectory to say that for some, ghosts and demons haunt the emptied space where ancestors, murdered in soul or body, once lived.

References

Beckett, S. (1954). *Waiting for Godot.* New York, NY: Grove Press.
Benjamin, W. (1940). Theses on the Philosophy of History. In, H. Arendt, (Ed.) (1973). *Illuminations.* New York, NY: Shocken Press.
Butler, J. (2004). *Precarious Life: The Powers of Mourning and Violence.* London: Verso.
Faimberg, H. (1988). The Telescoping of Generations – Genealogy of Certain Identifications. *Contemp. Psychoanal.* 24:99–117.
Faimberg, H. (2005). *The Telescoping of Generations: Listening to the Narcissistic Links Between Generations.* New York, NY: Brunner-Routledge.
Ferenczi, S. (1909). Introjection and Transference. In *Sex in Psychoanalysis*, Charleston, SC: Bibliobazaar, 2009.
LaCapra, D. (2001). *Writing History, Writing Trauma.* Baltimore, MD: Johns Hopkins University Press.
Laplanche, J. (1989). *New Foundations for Psychoanalysis.* Oxford: Basil Blackwell.
Levy, R. (2012). From Symbolization to Non-Symbolizing within the Scope of a Link: From Dreams to Shouts of Terror Caused by an Absent Presence. *Int. J. Psychoanal.,* 93:837–862.
Loewald, H. (1979). The Waning of the Oedipus Complex. *J. Amer. Psychoanal. Assoc.,* 27:751-775.
O'Neill, E. (1956). *Long Day's Journal Into Night.* New Haven, CT: Yale University Press.

Index

9/11 memorial 7–8

abjection 145
Abraham, N. 3, 11, 39 n.5, 41 n.14, 106, 194
"absence-mindedness" 102, 111
absent presences 4, 19, 20, 25, 198, 201
Abuladze, Tengiz 193
abyss, working at the edge of 5
Aciman, Andre 132
affect 2, 80, 81, 163–6, 169–71, 173–4
agency 172–3
alienaction 100
alienated identifications 201
alien self 75
alien thoughts 53
aliveness, feelings of 24, 38
Althusser, Louis 180
Altman, N. 53
ambivalence 25, 38, 62, 103, 187
American Civil War 6
analysts' own ghosts 65–6, 87–8, 95, 115, 125–37, 140–7
analytic third 23, 49
ancestors: enacted dimensions 76–81; energy for present-day living 70; ghosts as reluctant ancestors 19–45; ghosts becoming ancestors 68–70, 73, 77–8, 88, 146
Angel of History, The (Benjamin, 1940) 200
angels 109, 200
anger, repressed 164–5
Ann (case study) 80–9
Antigone 193
anti-psychoanalysis 109
anti-Semitism 126, 128, 131, 135

anxiety 81
archaic objects 149
area of omnipotence 30
Arendt, Hannah 133, 179, 193
Arica, Y. 50
Aron, L. 126
Aronson, Seth 131
Arzy, S. 53
Askara 54
asylum patients 8
Atlas, G. 47, 49
attachment 25, 29, 47, 55, 163–6, 175
attunement of significant other 163–6, 175
Atwood, G. 161, 162, 163, 164
Auerhahn, N. C. 71, 75
aura 99, 101, 108
authority 21, 23, 155–6, 193
Avedon, Richard 98, 117

Bach, S. 30
bad-me 53
Bandura, A. 172
Baranger, M. 3, 32, 152
Baranger, W. 3, 32, 152
Barthes, R. 4, 101, 108, 111
Beckett, Samuel 199
Benjamin, J. 3, 47, 49, 55, 56
Benjamin, Walter 93, 101, 108, 109, 183–4, 190, 200
Beratis, S. 32
Bergmann, M. 28, 129
Bion, W.R. 4–5, 19, 30, 39 n.1, 64
Bitov, Andrei 188
Blessing, J. 107
blind spots 129

body: of analyst 21–3, 30, 32–3; body ego 30–1, 33; bringing terror 113–14; disembodiment 23, 113–14; embodiment 6, 21–3, 30, 31–6, 74, 199 *see also* somaticity
Bollas, C. 2, 26, 33–4, 39 n.3, 39 n.5
Bolognini, S. 21, 39 n.3
Bonowitz, C. 115
boundaries, professional 13, 140–7
Bowlby, J. 175
Boyarin, D. 126
Bracken, K. 8
bracketing 35
Brandchaft, B. 168–9
breasts 83–4, 113–14, 198
bridge worlds 5
Bromberg, P. 29, 39 n.5, 53, 95
burials 185
Burke, Edmund 183, 194
Busch, F. 28
Butler, J. 147, 201

Carmilla (Le Fanu, 1871) 90 n.10
Caruth, C. 2, 93, 100, 111, 112, 113, 115, 116, 117
Cassidy, J. 175
Catholicness 66–7
Charlie (case study) 19–45
Chasidic tradition 46, 50–1, 53
Chasseguet-Smirgel, Janine 136
childhood trauma 19–20, 115, 129, 163–6, 169
cinema and film 7, 24, 72, 74, 88, 191–4
Civil War, American 6
clinical impasse 5, 11, 65, 117, 153, 170–1
collective amnesia 183
collective nostalgia 183
collusion 49
colonization 65
communism 145, 155, 179–81, 182
companion volume 1, 9–10
conflict theory 126
confusion of tongues 38, 41 n.13, 48–9
containment 55–6
contamination of others 21, 22, 49
continuum, trauma on a 9, 26, 71, 76
Corrigan, E. 56
cultural amnesia 183
culture 12–14

Dagan, H. 54
Daniel, Julii 187
Danny (case study) 46, 47–58
Davis, D. B. 159, 176
Davoine, F. 3, 5, 7
Dawson, Anthony 172–3
Day Watch (2004) 192–3
"dead mother" 35, 48, 55, 60, 172, 174–6
death: Death Drive 137; death in life 4; group of authors affected by 2; knowing the difference between life and death 111–13; preoccupation with dying 20, 31; and present absences 2; space between life and death 93–122, 188–90
debt to the dead 186, 194
defensive/protective mechanisms 71
Delia (slave) 160–1
demons, definitions of 3
depersonalization 148, 151, 154
depression 61–2, 65, 66, 164, 174
Derrida, J. 96, 179–81, 184, 194–5
Deutsch, R. 2
developmental trauma 19–20, 163–6, 169
Dimen, M. 141, 142, 144
disavowal 3, 19
disavowed vampires 11
disembodiment 23, 113–14
disorganized state 166
disorientation 148
dissociation: alienated identifications 201; and defensive/protective mechanisms 71; and the fear of contamination 49; ghosts 27–8; identifying in analytic treatment 72–3; integration as opposite to 86; and not-me 72, 73; not-me 53, 56; and rage 164, 165; repressed ghosts versus dissociated vampires 76; trauma and desymbolized somatic ghosts 29–31; and vampires 11, 27, 70–1, 72–3, 74–6
dissociative identity disorder 71, 75
divorce 47
doppelgängers 9, 24
Douglass, Frederick 166, 167–8
Dracula (Stoker, 1897) 90 n.10
draugrs 24
dreams: analysis as induced dreaming 4; Ann (case study) 82; and the enacted dimension 79; indicating resurgence of

ghosts 37; as 'not-me' experiences 53; and totalitarian objects 149–50
dybbuks 3, 11, 24, 46–58, 50–1
dying, preoccupation with 20, 31
dysregulation 47

early trauma theory 115, 129 *see also* childhood trauma
eating disorders 60
ego: beliefs 156; Charlie (case study) 28, 30; Richard (case study) 64; totalitarian objects 148, 149, 151–5
Ego Psychologists 129, 131
Eliade, M, 118 n.2
embodiment 6, 21–3, 30, 31–6, 74, 199
emptiness 148–9, 175, 177, 198, 201
enacted dimensions: alienated identifications 201; dissociated vampires 76–92; negative enactment 109–11; somaticity 19, 31–6; specter of the Shoah 135
enactive memory 78, 79
encrypted identification 3, 11–12
Engels, Friedrich 145
enigmatic messages 108
ephemerality 96, 108
Epic of Gilgamesh, The 24
Erikson, Erik 151, 154, 155
Eros 3, 10–11, 59, 60, 61, 64, 67, 198–9
evil, presence of 20, 50
excess 47, 55–6
excommunication of ghosts 50–1
exile 129–30, 132, 186
exorcism 50
experiential insight 79

facilitating environments 101
Faimberg, H. 3, 75, 201
fainting 20–2, 26, 35
Falzeder, E. 143
Farhi, N. 102, 111
fathers: analysts' own 111, 112, 127–9, 173–4; Ann (case study) 84, 85; Danny (case study) 47–50; and developmental trauma 164–5; losses passed down via parents 76; "Matin"/ "Martin with an (a)" (case study) 95, 106, 111, 112; and totalitarian objects 156–7
fear 20, 29, 49, 51

Felman, S. 116
Fenichel, Otto 130–1, 149, 153
Ferenczi, Sandor 7, 21, 41 n.13, 143, 201
Ferris, A. 105–6
Ferro, A. 4, 32
film and cinema 7, 24, 72, 74, 88, 191–4
Fineman, M. 98
Fiscalini, J. 28
folklore 72–3, 74
Fonagy, P. 39 n.5, 75
fort/da game 103–4
fragmented self 129
Fraiberg, S. 40 n.9
Frankenberg, R. 163
Freedman, N. 28, 40 n.10
Freud, Anna 134
Freud, Sigmund: the body 32; conflict theory 126; Death Drive 137; early trauma theory 115; ego 28, 30, 74; evenly hovering attention 4; fort/da game 103–4; ghosts 3, 89 n.1; melancholia/melancholy 2, 10, 28, 147; *nachtraglikeit* 29; the occult 7; "political Freudians" 130; professional ghosts 12–13; religion 153; shadow of the object 26, 28; and totalitarian objects 156; the uncanny 24, 149
Friedman, L. 126
Fromm, Erich 126–7
Fromm. M. G. 75
future already present 6

Gaines, R. 8, 29
Gampel, Y. 3
gaps, closing of 95
gaps in narrative 2
García Márquez, Gabriel 187
Gaudilliere, J.M. 3, 7
Geller, Mikhail 182
genetic programme 154
Gerson, Sam 1–2, 3, 11, 49, 66, 174, 176, 177
gestalts 151–2
Ghent, E. 114
"ghosting" 9, 10, 11
ghosts: analysts' own ghosts 65–6, 87–8, 115, 125–37, 140–7; in the consulting room 11–12, 19–45; definitions of 1–4, 19, 24–9, 47; in

folklore 72–3, 74; ghost pictures 105–6; good ghosts 40 n.8; haunting the profession 12–13; as iconic 185; impactful presence of ghosts 3; as internalization gone awry 19, 64; in Jewish tradition 54; and loss 28–9; media portrayals 8; metabolization of ghosts 11, 35; modern-day proliferation of 9; phantom fathers 106; popular culture 6–8, 69; in psychoanalytic literature 69; recognition versus justice 195; as reluctant ancestors 19–45; in Russia 185; spectral bond 30–1; in the superego position 61, 64; as unmetabolized objects 11, 20, 23, 63–4; what does the ghost want from me 198 *see also* dybbuks; vampires
Gods and God-like figures 149, 153, 154
Gogol, Nikolai 189, 190
golem 140, 143, 146
goners 190
good-me 53
Gordon, P. 56
Gottlieb, R. M. 74
grandparents: analysts' own 66, 131–2; Marissa (case study) 169–71; Richard (case study) 60; third generation transmission 76, 81–2
Grand, S. 3, 32, 75
Green, Andre 35, 48, 100, 149, 174
Grossman, Vassily 181
Grotstein, James 5
guilt 135, 137
gulags 179–81, 186, 187, 193
Gump, J. 166

Habermas, Jürgen 181
Hambourg, M. 98
Harris, A. 2, 4, 5, 23, 26, 31, 65–6, 67, 117, 144, 146–7
Hartman, J.J. 55
haunted, need for words such as 7
haunting, in analytic work 72
hauntology 180–1, 195
Heimann, Paula 134
Herman, C. 143
Himes, M. 97
Hinshelwood, R.D. 156

Historikerstreit 181
history: being a victim of 66; historicization of psychoanalysis 125, 131; historicization of Soviet terror 191; historicization of the Holocaust 181; History versus history 67; interpretation of 184–5, 187; long hand of history 7
Holocaust: Ann (case study) 81–9; compared to slavery 174, 175; compared to Soviet terror 179, 181, 182, 184; Richard (case study) 66; spectre of 7, 129, 131–3, 199
home 118 n.3
homosexuality 61, 64, 127

id 151–2
idealization 3, 64, 67, 152–154
identification 33, 41, 48, 76, 84, 111, 113, 116, 183; alienated identifications 201; encrypted identification 3, 11–12; projective identification 64, 135; radioactive identification 3
impasse, clinical 5, 11, 65, 117, 153, 170–1
impasse in mourning 23
incest 143, 146
integration, as opposite to dissociation 86
intergenerational trauma: Charlie (case study) 35–6; dissociation 75–6; and ghosts 3; Holocaust 132; sexual boundary violation 142–3; slavery 159–78; transmission mechanisms 176–8; zones of non-symbolization 200–1
internalization 11, 19, 25–7, 33, 64
internal objects, repair of 5–6, 65
internet 9
interpersonalism 25
interpretation 40, 62, 77–78, 101, 108, 114–115, 134, 184, 189
interpsychic-intersomatic transmission 22, 31–6
interpsychic space 11, 21, 26, 78, 89 n.2
interruption 117
intersubjectivity 39 n.3, 56, 112, 163, 171
intrapsychic 1, 23, 28, 32, 35, 66, 127, 131, 153
Iofe, Veniamin 182, 184

Jacobs, Lynne 162
Jacobson, Edith 131

Jacoby, Russell 130
Jacovy, M. 129
Jewish identity 46, 54, 66–7, 125–37
Jordan, W. 176
Jung, C. 143
justice 194–5

Katz, G. 19, 25, 27, 31, 39 n.3, 69, 79
Keller, C. 94, 103, 107
Kestenberg, J. 129
Kestenberg, M. 129
Klee, Paul 200
Klein, Melanie 135, 137
Kohut, Heinz 127–9
Kohut, Thomas 127–9, 136–7
Krauss, R. 106
Kris, Anton 127, 130–1
Kris, Ernst 127
Kuriloff, E. 127, 132, 133, 134, 135

Lacan, Jacques 143
LaCapra, D. 111, 201
Langer, Lawrence 184
language: expansion of vocabulary 10–11; language action 78, 79–80; naming 96–8; and trauma 93–4
LaPlanche, J. 47, 108, 198
Laub, D. 71, 75, 112, 116
Levine, H. 115
Levy, R. 200
Leys, R. 112
Likhachev, Dmitry 186
Liliths 54
liminality 98–116, 129, 149
Lin, Maya 7
listening 94
Little, Margaret 6
The Living (Veledinsky, 2006) 193–4
Lockot, Regine 132–6
Loewald, H. 3, 201; daylight of analysis 73, 88; definitions of ghosts 47; and the enacted dimension 77–8, 79–80; ghosts becoming ancestors 5, 68–70, 73, 77–8, 88, 146; internalization 33; interpsychic-intersomatic space 21, 24–8, 35, 38, 39 n.3; language action 79–80; Oedipal trajectory 201; repressed ghosts versus dissociated vampires 11; unmetabolized objects 64
Lombardi, R. 117
Long Day's Journey Into Night (O'Neill) 199
long hand of history 7
loss 2–3, 8, 10, 13, 26, 28, 35–8, 47, 61, 63, 74, 96, 107, 111, 114, 126, 128, 132, 137, 143, 147, 164, 174, 180, 185, 188, 190, 199, 201
Lost 8
love 28–9, 59–60, 62, 65, 67, 84
Lukianenko, Sergei 192
Luria, Rabbi Isaac 50

Maccoby, M. 127
madness 20, 21
mafia objects 151, 152
Magical Realism 187
Makari, G. 143
malignant 20, 33, 38
Mantel, H. 98
Marissa (case study) 169–70
Marx, Karl 145, 179–81
masculinity, fear of 49
masturbation 54, 55
"Matin"/"Martin with an (a)" (case study) 95–118
McCarthy, Joe 130
McGleughlin, J. 117
media portrayals 8
medicalization of psychoanalysis 130
melancholia/melancholy 4, 10, 11; and absent presence 201; Freud on 2, 10, 28, 147; intractable melancholia 10; into mourning 6, 147; post-revolutionary 180, 194; un-knowledge 2; *Zero City* (Shakhnazarov, 1988) 192
Melville, H. 101
memory: bodily memory 114; and childhood trauma 20; collective amnesia 183, 184; enactive memory 78; false memory syndrome 144; and ghosts 185; historical memory 66, 184–5; memorials 7–8; memories-in-action 28; petrification 31; re-living the past versus remembering 79; reminiscences 28, 32; repetition of the past 146; and sexual life 191

mentalize 40, 129, 135
metabolization of ghosts 11, 35, 63
metaphor 180
Michaels, W. B. 117
migration 81, 83, 128, 129–31
Milner, Marion 101
mind object 56
mirrors 98, 99, 115
Mitscherlich, Alexander 137
Mitscherlich, Margarete 137
Morrison, Toni 171
mothers: analysts' 52; Ann (case study) 82; Charlie (case study) 27; "dead mother" 35, 48, 55, 60, 172, 174–6; depression of 65; and developmental trauma 164–5, 166, 169–71; internalizations of 27; losses passed down via parents 76; Marissa (case study) 169–71; "Matin"/"Martin with an (a)" (case study) 95, 99, 101; Richard (case study) 60, 64–5; and slavery 168; and totalitarian objects 156–7; as tyrants 149
mourning: communal experiences of 185; cultural genres of 179; disrupted mourning 29; and guilt 137; impasse in mourning 23; inabilities to mourn 181–3; and justice 194–5; marking passage from life to death 113; and melancholy 2, 6, 11, 147; mimetic mourning 187; political theory of 183–5; and sexual abuse 147; in socialist Russia 182, 185; stuckness in 10; unmourned object loss 63, 74
multiple personality disorders 71
de M'Uzan, M. 149, 154

nachtraglikeit 29
Naiburg, S. 94
nameless dread 19, 20, 29, 30, 34
naming 94, 96–8, 100
narcissism 128–9, 137, 156
narrative: as antidote to haunting 10, 14; ghost storytelling 189–90; versus interpsychic-intersomatic transmission 34; and present absences 2; redemptive narrative 184
Nazis 125–6, 130, 135, 155, 179, 181–3
negative enactment 94, 112

negative, study of the 149
neutral analyst 30
Nguyen, L. 100, 118
Night Watch (2004) 192–3
Nolte, Ernst 181
nonbeing states 93–118
non-present 155–6
nonverbal transmssions: Ann (case study) 82; and archaic objects 149; Charlie (case study) 22, 23, 30, 33; and the enacted dimension 78, 80, 114–16; intergenerational trauma 84
Norris, Stephen M. 197 n.35
nothing, transmission of 177 *see also* emptiness
not-me 47, 53, 56, 151

obesity 31
object representations 26–7
occult 7
Ogden, T. 2, 29
omnipotence 30, 65, 98
O'Neill, Eugene 199
opacity 22
original creations 78–9

parents *see* fathers; intergenerational trauma; mothers
partial identities 151
past-as-present re-eruptions 28
patriarchy 143
personal ideologies 152
personality, assimilation into 64, 69, 70, 73, 78
petrification 31
Phelan, P. 104, 107, 109, 110
photographs 94, 98, 102–7, 108–9, 114
Poland, W. S. 78
Pontalis, J. B. 94, 108, 112, 113
popular culture 6–8, 69, 72–3, 159, 196 n.18
portrait making 98, 104
preconsciousness 149
pre-Oedipal attachment 64, 65, 66–7, 84, 129
present absences 1–2, 94, 109, 155–6, 174 *see also* "dead mother"

preverbal development phase 30, 36
projection 64
projective identification 64, 135
Proust, Marcel 73, 78
psychiatric patients 8
psychoanalytic profession 8, 69, 125–37, 140–7
psychosomatic illness 132
psychotic core 20
Puget, J. 3, 153
punctum 111, 117

Quinn, S. 129

racism 162, 173
Racker, Heinrich 4
radioactive identification 3
Raymond, C. 103, 104, 105, 109
recognition 27, 35, 38, 39, 41, 46, 70, 87, 90, 91, 92, 94, 101, 107, 130, 165, 205, 209
redemptive narrative 184
Reed, G. 115
reenactment 26, 28, 31–6
reflection 99–100
Reis, B. 3
religion 127, 153–4 *see also* Jewish identity
re-living the past 79
reminiscences 28, 32
repair of internal objects 5–6, 65
Repentance (Abuladze, 1984) 193–4
repetition 26, 146
repressions 27–8, 70, 71, 72, 76
retraumatization 73
retributive justice 195
Rey, Henri 65
Rey, J.H. 5
Richard (case study) 59–68
Rosenblum, R. 29
Rosenfeld, Herbert 151, 152, 153
Rothe, Katarina 135
Roudinesco, Elisabeth 180
Rozanov, Vasily 191
Russia 181–95

sadism 136, 137
saving objects 148–57

Schafer, Roy 65
Šebek, M. 148, 152–3
Secret, Le 7
secrets 22, 25, 28, 53, 208
self holding 35
self-regulation, failure of 56
sense of self 168–74
sensorimotor level 80
sexual abuse 19–20, 74–5
sexuality 84
sexual life: Charlie (case study) 31; Danny (case study) 48, 49, 53–5, 56–7; and memory 191; Richard (case study) 61; sexual boundary violation 140–7
shadow life of ghosts 28
shadow of the other 9
Shakhnazarov, Karen 191
Shalamov, Varlam 182
shame 53, 55–6, 59, 66–8, 135, 164
Shengold, L. 29
Shoah *see* Holocaust
Siniavsky, Andrei 186–7, 188–91
sins 47, 51, 52, 54, 56
Sinsheimer, K. 2
situational illness 33–4, 67
Skype sessions 23, 49
slavery 13, 159–78
Slavin, M.O. 117
Slochower, J.A. 8, 35
Smith, H.F. 27
Smith, S. 74
Socarides, D. D. 163
socialism 179–95
Solzhenitsyn, Alexander 181
somaticity 6; in analyst 19, 20–1; Ann (case study) 81, 82–3; interpersonal/relational aspects of 32; interpsychic-intersomatic transmission 31–6; trauma and desymbolized somatic ghosts 29–31; vampires 80 *see also* enacted dimensions
soul murder 29
Soviet Union 179–95
spectral bond 30–1
spiritism 6–7
split-off self state 75, 83, 129, 153
Starr, K. 126
Stein, R. 47
Stern, D. 26, 39 n.5

Stolorow, R. 31, 100, 112, 161, 162, 163, 164
Strozier, Charles 127
St. Vincent Millay, E. 101
subjectivity: of analyst 2, 125, 135; intersubjectivity 39 n.3, 56, 112, 163, 171; and slavery 161, 166–74; trans-subjective area 153–4
subjugation 166–8, 170, 171
suicide 29, 37–8, 109–10
Sullivan, Harry Stack 53
Sundell, M. 103
superego 61, 64, 133, 151–2, 153
survival patterns 149, 154
survivor guilt 35–6
symbolization 29, 36, 43, 54, 57, 81, 92, 94, 105, 106, 111, 129, 214, 216

telescoping of generations 3
testimony 94, 120, 127, 134
Thanatos 3, 10–11, 198, 199
third generation transmission 76, 81–2
Thirdness 3
third, the analytic 23, 49
thought transference 7
"too muchness" 47, 55–6
Torok, M. 3, 11, 39 n.5, 41 n.14, 106, 194
totalitarianism 156, 179
totalitarian objects 13, 148, 149–57
totality and wholeness 151–2
Tottman, N. 107
Townsend, C. 102, 103
transference-countertransference: action and reflection 144; and the analyst 67; Ann (case study) 86; Charlie (case study) 22, 25, 33–4; enacted dimensions 78–9; of ghosts 2, 24; ghosts and vampires in the matrix 77–8; ghosts becoming ancestors 70; and neutrality 30; reenactment 32; saving objects 148; totalitarian objects 148–57; transference neurosis 77–9
transfiguration 32
transitional spaces 101
trans-subjective area 153–4
trauma: absent presences 201; childhood trauma 19–20, 115, 129, 163–6, 169; and context 162; continuum of 9, 26, 71, 76; definitions of 162; developmental trauma 19–20, 163–6, 169; Freud's early trauma theory 115–16; historical memory versus psychic damage 66; as interaction between psyche and environment 71; and language 94; in liminal spaces 129; naming 100; and nonbeing 93–4, 116; risks of speaking aloud about 29; and slavery 161, 162–6; Trauma versus trauma 27–8, 29–31, 40 n.9, 71, 76; unsymbolizable trauma 72 *see also* intergenerational trauma

uncanny prescience 2
uncanny, the 7, 24, 30, 143–4, 148, 149; and dreams 151; in the grave 185; and Soviet terror 193–4; and totalitarian objects 153–4
uncertainty, basic 148–57
unconscious: archaic objects 149; communication 7; dynamic versus descriptive 70; and nonbeing 93–4; and preconscious interplay 25; transmission 25; vampire tastes blood in analyst's recognition 78, 87
undeadness 10; Charlie (case study) 19, 21, 31; as cost of surviving trauma 36; and fainting 35; laying to rest in the enacted dimension 76–81; vampires as dissociated trauma 73
underinternalizations 26, 33
unintegration 101, 163, 165
unknowable, the 94
un-knowledge 2
unmetabolized objects, ghosts as 11, 20, 23, 63–4
unmourned object loss 74
un-patients 38
unthought 40, 42, 44, 53, 115, 132, 133, 181
unwelcoming feelings 21

vampires 3; analysts' own 87–8; Ann (case study) 80–9; Charlie (case study) 31, 35, 37–8; dead-undead dyad 21; definitions of 24–9; in folklore 72–3, 74; and the Holocaust 82–3;

intergenerational trauma 75–6; and loss 28–9; media portrayals 8; in psychoanalytic literature 69; repressed ghosts versus dissociated vampires 11, 27, 71–2; and sexual abuse 74–5; and sexuality 31; and Siniavsky 189, 190; and Soviet terror 189, 190, 192; as subset of ghosts 27; unmourned object loss 74; vampires that menace 69–92; vampiric shadows 29
Vartzopoulos, I. 32
Verdery, Katherine 185
Vietnam War 7
violence 17, 29, 30, 36, 44, 62, 128, 156, 167, 176, 201, 212, 214
visual register 114–16
Vital, Rabbi Chaim 50
vocabulary, expansion of 10–11
Vonnegut, Kurt 146

Waiting for Godot (Beckett) 199
war, long shadow of 6–8

Welles, J.K. 31
"When the Third is Dead" (Gerson, 2009) 1
wholeness 151–2, 155
Winnicott, D. W. 30, 56, 65, 101, 115
Winterson, J. 95
witnessing 1–2, 3, 140; as antidote to haunting 10, 14; failure of 2; and naming 100; vampires 86; verbal 30
Woodman, Francesca 94, 102–7, 108–9, 114, 117
words 22, 23, 29–30
World War I 6
World War II 7
Wrye, H.K. 31

Yakovlev, Aleksandr 181
Yassa, M. 74
Yetman, N. R. 160, 172, 173

Zero City (Shakhnazarov, 1988) 191–2
zombies 24

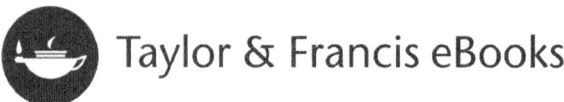

Taylor & Francis eBooks

Helping you to choose the right eBooks for your Library

Add Routledge titles to your library's digital collection today. Taylor and Francis ebooks contains over 50,000 titles in the Humanities, Social Sciences, Behavioural Sciences, Built Environment and Law.

Choose from a range of subject packages or create your own!

Benefits for you
- Free MARC records
- COUNTER-compliant usage statistics
- Flexible purchase and pricing options
- All titles DRM-free.

Benefits for your user
- Off-site, anytime access via Athens or referring URL
- Print or copy pages or chapters
- Full content search
- Bookmark, highlight and annotate text
- Access to thousands of pages of quality research at the click of a button.

REQUEST YOUR FREE INSTITUTIONAL TRIAL TODAY

Free Trials Available
We offer free trials to qualifying academic, corporate and government customers.

eCollections – Choose from over 30 subject eCollections, including:

Archaeology	Language Learning
Architecture	Law
Asian Studies	Literature
Business & Management	Media & Communication
Classical Studies	Middle East Studies
Construction	Music
Creative & Media Arts	Philosophy
Criminology & Criminal Justice	Planning
Economics	Politics
Education	Psychology & Mental Health
Energy	Religion
Engineering	Security
English Language & Linguistics	Social Work
Environment & Sustainability	Sociology
Geography	Sport
Health Studies	Theatre & Performance
History	Tourism, Hospitality & Events

For more information, pricing enquiries or to order a free trial, please contact your local sales team:
www.tandfebooks.com/page/sales

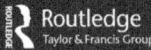

Routledge
Taylor & Francis Group

The home of Routledge books

www.tandfebooks.com